PEARSON

ALWAYS LEARNING

Clinical Medical Assistant
Student Workbook

Custom Edition for Condensed Curriculum International

Excerpts taken from:

*PowerPoint Slides to accompany Clinical Medical Assisting:
Foundations and Practice*
by Margaret Sc Frazier, Lori Ebert and Kristiana Sue Routh

Excerpts taken from:

PowerPoint Slides to accompany Clinical Medical Assisting: Foundations and Practice
by Margaret Sc Frazier, Lori Ebert and Kristiana Sue Routh
Copyright © 2008 by Pearson Education, Inc.
Published by Prentice Hall
Upper Saddle River, New Jersey 07458

Pearson Learning Solutions, 501 Boylston Street, Suite 900, Boston, MA 02116
A Pearson Education Company
www.pearsoned.com

Printed in the United States of America

8 9 10 V0CR 15 14

000200010271661534
RG

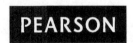

ISBN 10: 1-256-75220-7
ISBN 13: 978-1-256-75220-2

TABLE OF CONTENTS

PART A   CLINICAL MEDICAL ASSISTANT—STUDENT PACKET
          INFORMATION .... A-1 to A-60
PART B   CLINICAL MEDICAL ASSISTANT—STUDENT HANDOUTS ...... B-1 to B-48
PART C   CLINICAL MEDICAL ASSISTANT—SKILLS SUMMARY .... C-1 to C-10
PART D   CLINICAL MEDICAL ASSISTANT—STUDENT GRADUATE
          ASSISTANCE PACKET .... D-1 to D-20
PART E   CLINICAL MEDICAL ASSISTANT—PRESENTATION SLIDES ...... E-1 to E-58

PART A
Clinical Medical Assistant

STUDENT PACKET INFORMATION

TABLE OF CONTENTS

Topic   Page

Course Description A-3

Course Objectives A-4

Course Materials A-5

Expectations for the Student A-5

Teaching Methods Employed A-5

Evaluation and Grade Determination A-5

Course in Review A-7

Detailed Lesson Plans A-21

CLINICAL MEDICAL ASSISTANT PROGRAM

COURSE DESCRIPTION

This program prepares medical assistant students to perform patient clinical skills in various medical office settings. Students perform clinical procedures including administering medications, assisting with minor surgery, performing an electrocardiogram, obtaining laboratory specimens for testing, educating patients, and maintaining clinical equipment in an ambulatory care setting. Medical assistants perform routine clinical tasks to keep the offices of physicians, podiatrists, chiropractors, and optometrists running smoothly.

Clinical duties may include taking medical histories and recording vital signs, explaining treatment procedures to patients, preparing patients for examination, and assisting the physician during the examination. Medical assistants collect and prepare laboratory specimens or perform basic laboratory tests on the premises. They instruct patients about medication and special diets, prepare and administer medications as directed by a physician, authorize drug refills as directed, telephone prescriptions to a pharmacy, draw blood, prepare patients for x-rays, take electrocardiograms, and change dressings.

The Clinical Medical Assisting program is laid out in three sections:

Clinical Medical Assisting Section: Lessons #1–#14 covers the Clinical Medical Assisting section provides students with the knowledge and skills related to the medical office duties of the medical assistant. The Clinical Medical Assisting textbook is used for this section. The chapters on EKG and phlebotomy concepts are eliminated.

EKG Section: Lessons #15–#23 covers the specific knowledge and skills related to cardiovascular anatomy and physiology and performance of a 12-lead EKG test. Students learn how to accurately place leads onto the patient, run the EKG machine, perform basic measurements using the EKG strip, and identify normal tracings of the heart's electrical activity as well as identify common dysrhythmias. A separate EKG textbook and workbook is used for this section of the course.

Lab Services and Phlebotomy Section: Lessons #24–#40 provides the student with knowledge and skills related to collecting specimens for lab services including hematology, urinology, and other tests performed on body fluids. Students learn to perform a venipuncture procedure on adult, pediatric, and geriatric patients. A separate phlebotomy textbook and workbook is used for this section of the course.

COURSE OBJECTIVES

Upon completing this course, you will be able to:

- Explain the medical assistant's role in patient-centered care in various types of medical offices
- Describe how to prepare the office for a patient encounter
- Explain the concepts of medical and surgical asepsis
- Explain basic principles of pharmacology including how to administer various types of medication
- Explain how to measure vital signs
- Discuss how to help the physician in minor surgery including the identification of surgical supplies and equipment and maintaining a sterile field
- Explain effective communication strategies
- Explain the concepts of infection control, patient safety, OSHA blood borne pathogen standards, and body mechanics
- Demonstrate how to initiate, maintain, and discontinue a peripheral IV on a practice arm
- Discuss how a medical assistant can assist in a medical emergency
- Discuss how a medical assistant can assist the physician in the following medical specialties: ophthalmology and otolaryngology, dermatology, gastroenterology, urology and male reproduction, obstetrics and gynecology, pediatrics, orthopedic medicine, neurology and mental health, endocrinology, pulmonary medicine, cardiology, and geriatrics
- Discuss how a medical assistant should provide instruction in diagnostic procedures such as with diagnostic imaging, analysis of urine, phlebotomy, analysis of blood, and microbiology
- Demonstrate effective handwashing technique for the medical environment
- Demonstrate use of personal protective equipment in the medical environment
- Explain how to measure a patient for axillary crutches and how to instruct patients in their use
- Explain how to perform a surgical hand scrub and how to apply and remove sterile gloves
- Explain how to open a sterile pack
- Apply the basic electrophysiologic principles of cardiac conduction to the anatomy and physiology of the body
- Identify proper placement of leads to ensure an accurate and consistent EKG reading
- Evaluate various EKG rhythm strips following established normal criteria for each of the wave forms and intervals
- Analyze a variety of EKG rhythm strips, identifying rate, rhythm and intervals
- Analyze a variety of EKG rhythm strips for common dysrhythmias
- Perform a 12-lead EKG test
- Explain the steps in selected specimen collection procedures performed by the phlebotomy technician
- Explain the safety procedures in performing specimen collection procedures
- Identify specific supplies and equipment used in selected specimen collection procedures
- Explain precautions and guidelines when collecting specimens in special populations such as pediatrics and geriatrics
- Define quality of care and explain the impact on patient medical care when quality and safety are compromised in phlebotomy procedures
- Perform a venipuncture on a variety of patient types

COURSE MATERIALS

Title: *Clinical Medical Assisting: Foundations and Practice*
Author: Margaret Schell Frazier and Connie Morgan

Title: *EKG Technician Program Standard,* Custom Edition
Author: Karen M. Ellis

Title: *EKG Technician Program Standard Student Workbook,* Custom Edition
Author: CCI

Title: *Phlebotomy Handbook: Blood Specimen Collection from Basic to Advanced,* 8th Edition
Author: Diana Garza and Kathleen Becan-McBride

Title: *Phlebotomy Technician Program Student Workbook*
Author: CCI

EXPECTATIONS FOR THE STUDENT

1. Students are expected to arrive for class on time

2. Absent students must contact their instructor prior to class time

3. Absent students will be expected to make up missed class work/assignments on their own time

4. Students will follow the rules and regulations of the facility

5. No student shall disrupt a class or interfere with the session or the learning or the other students

6. The Instructor will be the student's contact for all academic questions or concerns

7. Cell phones and pagers are to be turned off or to the vibrator mode while in class

8. Any student participating in any act of academic dishonesty, such as cheating, plagiarism, or collusion will be considered for dismissal from the program. Once dismissed, no condition of re-entrance will be considered.

TEACHING METHODS EMPLOYED

Lecture, class discussion, group discussions, role-playing, critical thinking exercises, and application activities related to the pharmacy. This course also includes hands on instruction in a variety of modalities.

EVALUATION AND GRADE DETERMINATION

Student performance will be evaluated utilizing the following analysis:
Attendance and class participation (50%)
- Quizzes (25%)
- Final Exam (25%)

It is vital that each student recognize that this class is a **pass/fail** class with **no** exceptions.

This Packet and any attachments are the confidential property of CCI and are for class purposes only – do not print

COURSE IN REVIEW

CLINICAL MEDICAL ASSISTANT SECTION: LESSONS #1–#14 . . . . A-21

LESSON #1: The Medical Assistant Profession and Health Care & Interpersonal
        Communications A-21

Textbook Reading:	Chapter #1 (pp. 1–13) and Chapter #2 (pp. 14–26) in *Clinical Medical Assisting: Foundations and Practices*
Slides:	Slides E 4–8
Homework:	Read Chapters #3 and #4
	Complete Chapter Review from Chapters #1 (pp. 12–13) & #2 (p. 25)

LESSON #2: Patient-Centered Care & Considerations of Extended Life A-22

Textbook Reading:	Chapter #3 (pp. 27–35) and Chapter #4 (pp. 36–46) in *Clinical Medical Assisting: Foundations and Practices*
Slides:	Slides E 9–13
Homework:	Read Chapters #5, #6, and #7.
	Complete Chapter Review from Chapters #3 (pp. 34–35) and #4 (pp. 45–46).

LESSON #3: The Clinical Environment A-23

Textbook Reading:	Chapter #5 (pp. 48–59), Chapter #6 (pp. 60–77), and Chapter #7 (pp. 78–94) in *Clinical Medical Assisting: Foundations and Practices*
Slides:	Slides E 14–21
Lab:	Complete a Medical History Form
	Non-Sterile Gloving
Homework:	Read Chapters # 8 and #9.
	Complete Chapter Review from Chapters #5 (pp. 58–59), #6 (p. 76), and #7 (pp. 93–94).

LESSON #4: Surgical Asepsis, Pharmacology, and Medical Administration A-24

Textbook Reading:	Chapter #8 (pp. 95–115) and Chapter #9 (pp. 116–146) in *Clinical Medical Assisting: Foundations and Practices*
Slides:	Slides E 22–26
Homework:	Complete Chapter Review from Chapters #8 (pp. 114–115) and #9 (pp. 144–145).

LESSON #5: Lab A-25

Lab:	Demonstrate Withdrawing Medication from a Vial
	Preparation and Administration of Oral Medication
	Administration of a Subcutaneous Injection
	Administration of an Intramuscular Injection
Homework:	Read Chapters #10 and #11

LESSON #6: Vital Signs and Minor Surgery A-26

Textbook Reading:	Chapter #10 – pp. 147–175 and Chapter #11 – pp. 176–199 in *Clinical Medical Assisting: Foundations and Practices*
Slides:	Slides E 27–33
Homework:	Complete Chapter Review from Chapters #10 (pp. 174–175) and #11 (pp. 198–199).

LESSON #7: Lab **A-27**

Quiz:	Clinical Medical Assistant Quiz #1: Chapters 1, 2, 3, 4, 5, 6, 7, 8, & 9 in *Clinical Medical Assisting: Foundations and Practices*
Lab:	Obtain an Oral Temperature with an Electronic Thermometer
	Obtain Aural Temperature with a Tympanic Thermometer
	Perform a Radial Pulse Count
	Obtain an Apical Pulse Count
	Perform a Respiration Count
	Measure Blood Pressure
Homework:	Read Chapters #16 and #18.
	Note: Skip chapters #12, #13, #14, #15, and #17 in the CMA text as this is covered in the Phlebotomy and EKG section of the program.

LESSON #8: Medical Imaging, Pulmonology, and Pulmonary Testing **A-28**

Textbook Reading:	Chapter #16 (pp. 306–323) and Chapter #18 (pp. 363–385) in *Clinical Medical Assisting: Foundations and Practices*
Slides:	Slides E 34–37
Homework:	Read Chapters #19 and #20.
	Complete Chapter Review from Chapters #16 (pp. 322–323) and #18 (p. 384).

LESSON #9: EENT, Immunology, and Allergies **A-29**

Textbook Reading:	Chapter #19 (pp. 386–413) and Chapter #20 (pp. 414–425) in *Clinical Medical Assisting: Foundations and Practices*
Slides:	Slides E 38–39
Lab:	Measure Distance Visual Acuity with a Snellen chart
Homework:	Read Chapters #21 and #22.
	Complete Chapter Review from Chapters #19 (pp. 411–412) and #20 (pp. 424–425).

LESSON #10: Dermatology and Endocrinology **A-30**

Textbook Reading:	Chapter #21 (pp. 426–445) and Chapter #22 (pp. 446–456) in *Clinical Medical Assisting: Foundations and Practices*
Slides:	Slides E 40–41
Homework:	Read Chapters #23 and #24.
	Complete Chapter Review from Chapters #21 (pp. 444–445) and #22 (pp. 454–455).

LESSON #11: Emergency Care, Gastroenterology, and Nutrition **A-31**

Textbook Reading:	Chapter #23 (pp. 458–498) and Chapter #24 (pp. 499–528) in *Clinical Medical Assisting: Foundations and Practices*
Slides:	Slides E 42–46
Lab:	Demonstrate a Triangular Sling
Homework:	Read Chapters #25 and #26.
	Complete Chapter Review from Chapters #23 (p. 497–498) and #24 (pp. 527–528).

LESSON #12: Orthopedics, Physical Therapy, Obstetrics, and Gynecology **A-32**

Textbook Reading:	Chapter #25 (pp. 529–562) and Chapter #26 (pp. 563–588) in *Clinical Medical Assisting: Foundations and Practices*
Slides:	Slides E 47–49
Quiz:	Clinical Medical Assistant Quiz #2: Chapters 10, 11, 16, 18, 19, 20, 21, 22, 23, and 24
Homework:	Read Chapters #27 and #28.
	Complete Chapter Review from Chapters #25 (p. 561) and #26 (p. 587).

LESSON #13: Pediatrics and Neurology **A-33**

Textbook Reading:	Chapter #27(pp. 589–608) and Chapter #28 (pp. 609–626) in *Clinical Medical Assisting: Foundations and Practices*
Slides:	Slides E 50–51
Homework:	Read Chapters #29, #30, #31, and #32.
	Complete Chapter Review from Chapters #27 (pp. 607–608) and #28 (p. 625).

LESSON #14: Mental Health, Oncology, Geriatrics, and Alternative Medicine **A-34**

Textbook Reading:	Chapter #29 (pp. 627–643), Chapter #30 (pp. 644–654), Chapter #31 (pp. 655–665), and Chapter #32 (pp. 668–678) in *Clinical Medical Assisting: Foundations and Practices*
Slides:	Slides E 52–58
Homework:	Complete Chapter Review from Chapters #29 (pp. 642–643), #30 (pp. 653–654), #31 (p. 664), and #32 (p. 676).
	Read Chapters #1 and #2 in *EKG Technical Program Standard, Custom Edition*

EKG SECTION: LESSONS #15–#23 .... **A-35**

LESSON #15: Coronary Anatomy and Physiology and Electrophysiology **A-35**

Textbook Reading:	Chapter #1 (pp. 1–12) and Chapter #2 (pp. 13–33) in *EKG Technical Program Standard*
Slides:	Slides D 2–14
Quiz:	Clinical Medical Assistant Quiz #3: Chapters 25, 26, 27, 28, 29, 30, 31, and 32 in *Clinical Medical Assisting: Foundations and Practices* text
Homework:	Read Chapters #3 and #4.

LESSON #16: Lead Morphology and Placement/Technical Aspects of the EKG **A-36**

Textbook Reading:	Chapter #3 (pp. 35–46) and Chapter #4 (pp. 47–59) in *EKG Technical Program Standard*
Slides:	Slides D 15–30
Lab:	Introduction to the EKG Machine
	Patient Preparation and Safety
	12-Lead Placement
	Performing a 12-Lead EKG
	Obtaining a Blood Pressure
Homework:	Read Chapters #5 and #6.

LESSON #17: Calculating Heart Rate and Rhythm Strip Interpretation **A-37**

Textbook Reading:	Chapter #5 (pp. 61–72) and Chapter #6 (pp. 73–77) in *EKG Technical Program Standard*
Slides:	Slides D 31–37
Quiz:	EKG Quiz #1: Chapters 1, 2, 3, and 4
Homework:	Read Chapter #7.

LESSON #18: Rhythms Originating in the Sinus Node **A-38**

Textbook Reading:	Chapter #7 (pp. 79–98) in *EKG Technical Program Standard*
Slides:	Slides D 38–43
Lab:	Performing a 12-Lead EKG
Homework:	Read Chapters #8 and #9.

LESSON #19: Rhythms Originating in the Atria and AV Junction **A-39**

Textbook Reading:	Chapter #8 (pp. 99–119) and Chapter #9 (pp. 121–132) in *EKG Technical Program Standard*
Slides:	Slides D 44–53
Lab:	Performing a 12-Lead EKG
Homework:	Read Chapter #10.

LESSON #20: Rhythms Originating in the Ventricles and AV Blocks **A-40**

Textbook Reading:	Chapter #10 (pp. 133–155) and Chapter #11 (pp. 157–176) in *EKG Technical Program Standard*
Slides:	Slides D 54–68
Lab:	Performing a 12-Lead EKG
Quiz:	EKG Quiz #2: Chapters 5, 6, 7, 8, and 9
Homework:	Read Chapter #12.

LESSON #21: Rhythm Practice Strips **A-41**

Textbook Reading:	Chapter #12 (pp. 177–301) in *EKG Technical Program Standard*
Slides:	Slides D 69–79
Lab:	Performing a 12-Lead EKG
Homework:	Read Chapter #13.

LESSON #22: Artificial Pacemakers **A-42**

Textbook Reading:	Chapter #13 (pp. 303–317) in *EKG Technical Program Standard*
Slides:	Slides D 80–83
Lab:	Performing a 12-Lead EKG
Quiz:	EKG Quiz #3: Chapters 10, 11, and 12
Homework:	Read Chapter #14.

LESSON #23: Diagnostic Electrocardiography **A-43**

Textbook Reading:	Chapter #14 (pp. 319–346) in *EKG Technical Program Standard*
Slides:	Slides D 84–93
Lab:	Performing a 12-Lead EKG

PHLEBOTOMY SECTION: LESSONS #24–#40 . . . . A-44

LESSON #24: Phlebotomy Practice and Quality Assessment A-44

Textbook Reading:	Chapter #1 (pp. 1–38) and Appendix #1 (pp. 546–549) in *Phlebotomy Handbook*
Slides:	Slides D 2–9
Lab:	Performing a 12-Lead EKG
Homework:	Review and complete questions pp. 34–38.

LESSON #25: Communication, Computerization, and Documentation A-45

Textbook Reading:	Chapter #2 (pp. 39–80) and Appendix #4 pp. 556–558) in *Phlebotomy Handbook*
Slides:	Slides D 10–14
Homework:	Review and complete questions pp. 74–80

LESSON #26: Professional Ethics, Legal and Regulatory Issues, and Infection Control A-46

Textbook Reading:	Chapter #3 (pp. 81–99) and Chapter #4 (pp. 101–137) in *Phlebotomy Handbook*
Slides:	Slides D 15–24
Lab:	Donning and Removing Gloves Gowning, Masking, and Gloving Removal Isolation Gown, Mask, and Gloves
Homework:	Review and complete questions pp. 97–100 and 134–137.

LESSON #27: Safety and First Aid, Medical Terminology, and Anatomy and Physiology
of Organ Systems A-47

Textbook Reading:	Chapter #5 (pp. 138–157) and Chapter #6 (pp. 158–206) *Phlebotomy Handbook*
Slides:	Slides D 25–48
Homework:	Review and complete questions pp. 154–157 and 200–206.

LESSON #28: The Cardiovascular and Lymphatic Systems A-48

Textbook Reading:	Chapter #7 (pp. 207–248) in *Phlebotomy Handbook*
Slides:	Slides D 49–62
Quiz:	Phlebotomy Quiz #1: Chapters 1, 2, 3, 4, 5, and 6
Homework:	Review and complete questions pp. 244–248.

LESSON #29: Blood Collection Equipment A-49

Textbook Reading:	Chapter #8 (pp. 249–280) in *Phlebotomy Handbook*
Slides:	Slides D 63–70
Homework:	Review and complete questions pp. 277–280.

LESSON #30: Preanalytical Complications Causing Medical Errors in Blood Collection A-50

Textbook Reading:	Chapter #9 (pp. 281–300) in *Phlebotomy Handbook*
Slides:	Slides D 71–80
Homework:	Review and complete questions pp. 297–300.

LESSON #31: Venipuncture Procedures A-51

Textbook Reading:	Chapter #10 (pp. 301–362) *Phlebotomy Handbook*
Slides:	Slides D 81–105
Lab:	Preparing for the Patient Encounter
	Hand Hygiene and Gloving Technique
	Basics of Patient Identification
	Use of a Tourniquet and Vein Palpation
	Decontamination of the Puncture Site
	Performing a Venipuncture
	Syringe Method
Homework:	Review and complete questions pp. 356–362.

LESSON #32: Capillary Blood Specimens A-52

Textbook Reading:	Chapter #11(pp. 363–382) in *Phlebotomy Handbook*
Slides:	Slides D 106–115
Lab:	Acquiring a Capillary Blood Specimen (Skin Puncture) using a Retractable Safety Device
	Blood Smears/Films for Microscopic Slides
Homework:	Review and complete questions pp. 379–382.

LESSON #33: Specimen Handling, Transportation, and Processing A-53

Textbook Reading:	Chapter #12 (pp. 383–404) *Phlebotomy Handbook*
Slides:	Slides D 116–125
Lab:	Hands-On Venipuncture Practice
Homework:	Review and complete questions pp. 400–404.

LESSON #34: Pediatric and Geriatric Procedures A-54

Textbook Reading:	Chapter #13 (pp. 405–443) in *Phlebotomy Handbook*
Slides:	Slides D 126–141
Quiz:	Phlebotomy Quiz #2: Chapters 7, 8, 9, 10, 11, and 12
Lab:	Hands-On Venipuncture Practice
Homework:	Review and complete questions pp. 440–443.

LESSON #35: Point-of-Care Collections A-55

Textbook Reading:	Chapter #14 (pp. 444–464) in *Phlebotomy Handbook*
Slides:	Slides D 142–154
Lab:	Hands-On Venipuncture Practice
Homework:	Review and complete questions pp. 461–464.

LESSON #36: Arterial, Intravenous, and Special Collections A-56

Textbook Reading:	Chapter #15 (pp. 465–499) in *Phlebotomy Handbook*
Slides:	Slides D 155–170
Lab:	Site-Preparation for Blood Culture Collection
	Safety Butterfly Assembly
	Evacuated Tube System for Blood culture Collection
	After Blood Culture collection by the Previous Methods
	Radial ABG Procedure
Homework:	Review and complete questions pp. 496–499.

LESSON #37: Urinalysis, Body Fluid, and Other Specimens **A-57**

Textbook Reading:	Chapter #16 (pp. 500–522) in *Phlebotomy Handbook*
Slides:	Slides D 171–180
Lab:	Hands-On Venipuncture Practice
Homework:	Review and complete questions pp. 519–522.

LESSON #38: Drug Use, Forensic Toxicology, Workplace Testing, Sports medicine, and Related Areas .. **A-58**

Textbook Reading:	Chapter #17 (pp. 523–544) in *Phlebotomy Handbook*
Slides:	Slides D 181–186
Lab:	Hands-On Venipuncture Practice
Homework:	Review and complete questions pp. 541–544.

LESSON #39: Finding a Job and the Basics of Vital Signs **A-59**

Textbook Reading:	Appendix #2 (pp. 550–554) and Appendix #5 (pp. 559–569) in *Phlebotomy Handbook*
Slides:	Slides D 187-197
Quiz:	Phlebotomy Quiz #3: Chapters 13, 14, 15, 16, and 17
Lab:	Taking Oral Temperature
	Assessing Peripheral Pulse Rate
	Taking Blood Pressure
	Assessing Respiration Rate
Student Workbook:	Certification Exam Review: NHA—CCMA Study Guide
Homework:	Study for the Final Exam.

LESSON #40: CMAA Final Exam **A-60**

Quiz:	CMAA Final Exam

Clinical Medical Assistant

Clinical Medical Assisting Section
Lesson Plans
Lessons #1–14

LESSON #1: THE MEDICAL ASSISTANT PROFESSION AND HEALTH CARE & INTERPERSONAL COMMUNICATIONS

Textbook:
Clinical Medical Assisting: Foundations and Practices by Frazier and Morgan
Chapter #1: The Medical Assistant Profession and Health care, pp. 1–13
Chapter # 2: Interpersonal Communication, pp. 14–26

Objectives:
After completing this lesson, you should be able to:
- Define the medical assistant's role in the healthcare profession
- Explain the AMA's *Principles of Medical Ethics*
- Identify the professional characteristics of a medical assistant
- List the work responsibilities of a medical assistant
- Discuss the professional associations and their credentials for medical assistants
- Discuss verbal, nonverbal, nonverbal, and symbolic communication
- Discuss listening strategies
- Explain barriers to communication with patients
- Explain cultural and age factors as they relate to communication
- Explain the grief process

Handout:
Handout #1—What is HIPAA?
Handout #1a—Medical Terminology Study Notes

Student Slides:
Slides E 4–8

Lesson Topics:
This lesson covers the following topics.
- The History of Medicine
- Ethics and Patient Rights
- Professionalism
- Health-Care Team Members
- Medical Assistant Educational Programs
- Verbal Communication
- Nonverbal Communication
- Listening
- Developmental Stages of the Life Cycle
- Barriers to Communication
- The Grieving Process

Homework:
Complete the following assignments:
- Read Chapters #3 and #4.
- Complete Chapter Review from Chapters #1 (pp. 12–13) and #2 (p. 25).

LESSON #2: PATIENT-CENTERED CARE & CONSIDERATIONS OF EXTENDED LIFE

Textbook:

Clinical Medical Assisting: Foundations and Practices by Frazier and Morgan

Chapter #3: Patient-Centered Care, pp. 27–35

Chapter #4: Considerations of Extended Life, pp. 36–46

Objectives:

After completing this lesson, you should be able to:

- Define the medical assistant's role in patient-centered care
- Discuss wellness and the holistic approach to health care
- Explain the mind-body connection
- Describe the different types of pain, pain assessment, and pain management
- Discuss the methods of assisting patients with special needs
- Define the medical assistant's role as it relates to extended life and terminal care
- Discuss organ donation and transplant concepts
- Discuss advance medical directives and the durable power of attorney in health care
- Explain living wills and life-prolonging declarations
- Discuss hospice

Student Slides:

Slides E 9-13

Lesson Topics:

This lesson covers the following topics.

- Wellness
- A Holistic Approach to Health Care
- Pain
- Patients with Special Needs
- Organ and Tissue Donations
- Transplant Costs
- Organ and Tissue Donation Rules and Regulations
- Advance Medical Directives
- Hospice

Homework:

Complete the following assignments:

- Read Chapters #5, #6, and #7.
- Complete Chapter Review from Chapters #3 (pp. 34–35) and #4 (p. 46).

LESSON #3: THE CLINICAL ENVIRONMENT

Textbook:	*Clinical Medical Assisting: Foundations and Practices* by Frazier and Morgan

Chapter #5: The Clinical Environment and Safety in the Medical Office, pp. 48–59

Chapter #6: The Clinical Visit: Office Preparation and the Patient Encounter, pp. 60–77

Chapter #7: The Medical Asepsis, pp. 71–94

Objectives:
After completing this lesson, you should be able to:

- Define the medical assistant's role as it relates to safety in the medical office
- Discuss proper body mechanics for the medical office employee
- Describe procedures intended to provide a safe environment
- Discuss emergency plans for a medical facility
- Explain Standard Precautions and OSHA's Bloodborne Pathogen Standards
- Define the medical assistant's role in the clinical visit
- Define triage
- Discuss consent for treatment
- Discuss the medical record
- Describe the medical assistant's role in the promotion of infection control in the medical office
- Explain the cycle of infection and the body's natural defenses against infection
- Explain the practices related to aseptic technique for a health professional

Handout:
Handout #2: Common Abbreviations

Handout #3: History Form

Handout #4: Attachment "B"—Medical Record

Hands-On Lab Skills:
You will complete hands-on instruction in the following labs:

- Procedure #6–2: Complete a History Form
- Procedure #7: Non-Sterile Gloving

Lab Skills Discussion:
You will discuss the following hands-on skills in lab:

- Procedure #6–1: Prepare and Maintain the Medical Record
- Procedure #6–3: Document a Clinical Visit and Procedure
- Procedure #7–1: Hand Washing

Student Slides:
Slides E 14–21

Lesson Topics:
This lesson covers the following topics.

- Wellness
- A Holistic Approach to Health Care
- Pain
- Patients with Special Needs
- Organ and Tissue Donations
- Transplant Costs
- Organ and Tissue Donation Rules and Regulations
- Advance Medical Directives
- Hospice

Homework:
Complete the following assignments:

- Read Chapters #8 and #9.
- Complete Chapter Review from Chapters #5 (pp. 58–59), #6 (p. 76), and #7 (pp. 93–94).

LESSON #4: SURGICAL ASEPSIS, PHARMACOLOGY, AND MEDICAL ADMINISTRATION

Textbook: *Clinical Medical Assisting: Foundations and Practices* by Frazier and Morgan
Chapter #8: Surgical Asepsis, pp. 95–115
Chapter #9: Pharmacology and Medication Administration, pp. 116–146

Objectives: *After completing this lesson, you should be able to:*

- Differentiate between and explain the procedures for aseptic technique, sanitization, disinfection, and sterilization
- Discuss the medical assistant's role in administering and dispensing drugs
- Explain the basic actions and various types of effects of drugs in the body
- Explain how drugs are measured and conversions are calculated
- List safety guidelines that must be followed when drugs are administered
- Explain the various drug classifications
- Explain the legal guidelines for prescribing and administering controlled substances
- Identify and describe the forms and routes of drug administration

Handout: Handout #5: Body Mechanics

Lab Skills Discussion: *You will discuss the following hands-on skills in lab:*

- Procedure #8-1: *Sanitization*
- Procedure #8-2: Disinfection
- Procedure #8-3: Wrapping Surgical Instruments for Autoclave Sterilization
- Procedure #8-4: Loading and Operating an Autoclave
- Procedure #8-5: Opening a Sterile Surgical Pack to Create a Sterile Field
- Procedure #8-6: Using Transfer Forceps
- Procedure #8-7: Performing a Sterile Scrub (Surgical Hand Washing)
- Procedure #8-8: Sterile Gloving and Glove Removal
- Procedure #9-1: Demonstrate the Preparation of a Prescription for the Physician's Signature

Student Slides: Slides E 22–26

Lesson Topics: *This lesson covers the following topics.*

- Surgical Asepsis
- Sanitization, Disinfection, & Sterilization
- Wrapping Instruments and Preparing Sterile Trays
- Preparing the Surgical Field
- Alcohol-Based Hand Rubs
- Basic Pharmacology
- Medication Measurement and Conversion
- Safety Guidelines for Administering Medications
- The Prescription
- Forms and Routes for Medication Administration

Homework: *Complete the following assignments:*

- Complete Chapter Review from Chapters #8 (pp. 114–115) and #9 (pp. 144–145).

LESSON #5: LAB

Textbook:	*Clinical Medical Assisting: Foundations and Practices* by Frazier and Morgan
	N/A
Objectives:	*After completing this lesson, you should be able to:*
	• Complete lab skills as described in procedures
Handout:	Handout #6: Peripheral Intravenous
Lab skills Discussion:	*You will discuss the following hands-on skills in lab:*
	• Procedure #9-2: Demonstrate the Withdrawing Medication from an Ampule
	• Procedure #9-4: Demonstrate the Reconstitution of a Powdered Drug for Injection Administration
	• Procedure #9-5: Demonstrate the Administration of Medication during Infusion Therapy
	• Procedure #9-9: Demonstrate the Administration of a Z-Track Injection
Hands-On Lab Skills:	*You will complete hands-on instruction in the following labs:*
	• Procedure #9-3: Demonstrate Withdrawing Medication from a Vial
	• Procedure #9-6: Preparation and Administration of Oral Medication
	• Procedure #9-7: Administration of a Subcutaneous Injection
	• Procedure #9-8: Administration of an Intramuscular Injection
Lesson Topics:	*This lesson covers the following topics.*
	• Lab skills
Homework:	*Complete the following assignments:*
	• Read Chapters #10 and #11.

LESSON #6: VITAL SIGNS AND MINOR SURGERY

Textbook: *Clinical Medical Assisting: Foundations and Practices* by Frazier and Morgan
                     Chapter #10: Vital Signs, pp. 147–175

                     Chapter #11: Minor Surgery, pp. 176–199

Objectives: *After completing this lesson, you should be able to:*

- Explain the principles of vital signs and state the normal values for various age groups
- Explain the medical assistant's role in patient preparation, including gowning, positioning, draping, and office surgery
- Describe the methods of assessment used during a medical examination
- Explain the ways in which the medical assistant assists the physician during the medical examination
- List and describe surgeries performed in the medical office and how to set up the room for surgeries of the medical office
- Discuss preoperative, recovery, and postoperative care of the patient in the medical office
- Discuss the ways in which the MA assists the physician during minor surgery

Lab Skills Discussion: *You will discuss the following hands-on skills in lab:*

- Procedure #10-2: Obtain an Axillary Temperature with an Electronic Digital Thermometer
- Procedure #10-3: Obtain a Rectal Temperature with an Electronic Digital Thermometer
- Procedure #10-5: Obtain a Dermal Temperature with a Disposable Thermometer
- Procedure #10-10: Obtain Weight and Height Measurements
- Procedures #10-11: Demonstrate Patient Positions Used in a Medical Examination
- Procedures #10-12: Assist the Physician with the Physical Examination

Student Slides: Slides E 27–33

Lesson Topics: *This lesson covers the following topics.*

- Vital signs
- Preparing the Patient for a Physical Examination
- Assessment Methods Used in an Examination
- Surgeries Performed in the Medical Office
- Implied and Informed Consent
- Preoperative Care and Patient Preparation
- Assisting During Minor Surgery
- Recovery/Postoperative Care

Homework: *Complete the following assignments:*

- Complete Chapter Review from Chapters #10 (pp. 174–175) and #11 (pp. 198–199).

LESSON #7: LAB

Textbook:	*Clinical Medical Assisting: Foundations and Practices* by Frazier and Morgan
	N/A
Objectives:	*After completing this lesson, you should be able to:*

- Complete lab skills as described in procedures

Lab Skills Discussion: *You will discuss the following hands-on skills in lab:*

- Procedure #11-1: Prepare the Skin for Surgical Procedure
- Procedure #11-2: Set Up a Sterile Tray and Assist the Physician with Minor Surgical Procedures
- Procedure #11-3: Assist the Physician with Suturing
- Procedure #11-4: Assist the Physician with Suture or Staple Removal
- Procedure #11-5: Change a Sterile Dressing

Hands-On Lab Skills: *You will complete hands-on instruction in the following labs:*

- Procedure #10-1: Obtain an Oral Temperature with an Electronic Digital Thermometer
- Procedure #10-4: Obtain Aural Temperature with a Tympanic Thermometer
- Procedure #10-6: Perform a Radial Pulse Count
- Procedure #10-7: Obtain an Apical Pulse Count
- Procedure #10-8: Perform a Respiration Count
- Procedure #10-9: Measure Blood Pressure

Quiz/Test (Start of class):   Clinical Medical Assistant Quiz #1: Chapters 1, 2, 3, 4, 5, 6, 7, 8, & 9

Lesson Topics: *This lesson covers the following topics.*

- Lab Skills

Homework: *Complete the following assignments:*

- Read Chapters #16 and #18.

Note: Skip Chapters 12, 13, 14, 15, and 17 of the CMA textbook as this is covered in the Phlebotomy section of this program.

LESSON #8: MEDICAL IMAGING, PULMONOLOGY, AND PULMONARY TESTING

Textbook:

Clinical Medical Assisting: Foundations and Practices by Frazier and Morgan

Chapter #16: Medical Imaging, pp. 306–323

Chapter #18: Pulmonology and Pulmonary Testing, pp. 363–385

- *Note: Skip chapters #12, #13, #14, #15, and #17 in the CMA text as this is covered in the Phlebotomy and EKG section of the program.*

Objectives:

After completing this lesson, you should be able to:

- Define the medical assistant's role in medical imaging
- Describe the various medical imaging technologies and the information that can be obtained from each
- Identify safety guidelines that protect the patient and technician during radiographic procedures
- Discuss patient preparation, instructions, and positioning for various diagnostic imaging tests
- Define the medical assistant's role in a Pulmonology practice
- Discuss lung and chest mechanics and gas mechanics of respiration
- Describe the symptoms, causes, tests, and treatments of various pulmonary related diseases

Lab Skills Discussion:

You will discuss the following hands-on skills in lab:

- Procedure #16-1: Perform General Procedure for X-ray Examination
- Procedure #16-2: File and Loan Radiographic Records
- Procedure #18-1: Demonstrate Performance of Spirometry
- Procedure #18-2: Demonstrate Performance of Peak Flow Testing
- Procedure #18-3: Demonstrate Performance of the Mantoux Test by Intradermal Injection
- Procedure #18-4: Demonstrate patient Instruction in the Use of an Inhaler
- Procedure #18-5: Demonstrate patient Assistance in the Use of a Nebulizer

Student Slides:

Slides E 34–37

Lesson Topics:

This lesson covers the following topics.

- Radiology and Equipment
- Safety Precautions and Patient Protection
- Limited Scope Radiology
- Scheduling Radiographs
- Assisting with an X-ray
- Preparation of the X-ray Room
- Filing and Loaning Radiographic Records
- The Anatomy and Physiology of the Pulmonary System
- Diseases and Disorders of the Pulmonary System
- Pulmonary Assessment and Diagnosis
- Inhalers, Nebulizers, and Oxygen

Homework:

Complete the following assignments:

- Read Chapters #19 and #20.
- Complete Chapter Reviews from Chapters #16 (pp. 322–323) and #18 (p. 384).

LESSON #9: EENT, IMMUNOLOGY, AND ALLERGIES

Textbook:	*Clinical Medical Assisting: Foundations and Practices* by Frazier and Morgan
	Chapter #19: EENT, pp. 386–413
	Chapter #20: Immunology and Allergies, pp. 414–425
Objectives:	*After completing this lesson, you should be able to:*

- Define the medical assistant's role in the EENT office
- Describe the anatomy and physiology of the eye, ear, nose, nasal passages, and throat and associated diseases
- Discuss diagnostic procedures and assessments related to EENT
- Define the medical assistant' role in the immunology office
- Discuss the anatomy and physiology of the immune system
- List and describe immunodeficiency diseases and common autoimmune disorders

Lab Skills Discussion: *You will discuss the following hands-on skills in lab:*

- Procedure #19-2: Perform the Ishihara Color Vision Test
- Procedure #19-3: Perform Eye Irrigation
- Procedure #19-4: Perform Instillation of Eye Medication
- Procedure #19-5: Perform simple Audiometry
- Procedure #19-6: Perform Ear Irrigation
- Procedure #19-7: Perform Instillation of Ear Medication

Hands-On Lab Skills: *You will complete hands-on instruction in the following labs:*

- Procedure #19-1: Measure Distance Visual Acuity with a Snellen Chart

Student Slides: Slides E 38–39

Lesson Topics: *This lesson covers the following topics.*

- Anatomy, Physiology, Disorders, and Tests of the Ear
- Anatomy, Physiology, Disorders, and Tests of the Eye
- Anatomy, Physiology, Disorders, and Tests of the Nose and Throat
- Anatomy and Physiology of the Immune System
- Diseases and Disorders of the Immune system

Homework: *Complete the following assignments:*

- Read Chapters #21 and #22.
- Complete Chapter Reviews from Chapters #19 (pp. 411–412) and #20 (pp. 424–425).

LESSON #10: DERMATOLOGY AND ENDOCRINOLOGY

Textbook: *Clinical Medical Assisting: Foundations and Practices* by Frazier and Morgan
Chapter #21: Dermatology, pp. 426–445
Chapter #22: Endocrinology, pp. 446–456

Objectives: *After completing this lesson, you should be able to:*
- Define the medical assistant's role in the dermatology office
- List and describe common types of skin diseases and disorders
- Describe the medical assistant's role in the endocrinology office
- Discuss the anatomy and physiology of the endocrine system
- Discuss diseases and disorders of the endocrine system

Student Slides: Slides E 40–41

Lesson Topics: *This lesson covers the following topics.*
- The Anatomy and physiology of the Skin
- Diseases and Disorders of the Skin
- Cosmetic Treatment for Skin Conditions
- Anatomy and Physiology of the Endocrine System
- Endocrine Disorders

Homework: *Complete the following assignments:*
- Read Chapters #23 and #24.
- Complete Chapter Reviews from Chapters #21 (pp. 444-445) and #22 (pp. 454–455).

LESSON #11: EMERGENCY CARE, GASTROENTEROLOGY, AND NUTRITION

Textbook:	*Clinical Medical Assisting: Foundations and Practices* by Frazier and Morgan
	Chapter #23: Emergency Care, p. 458–498
	Chapter #24: Gastroenterology and Nutrition, pp. 499–528
Objectives:	*After completing this lesson, you should be able to:*

- Define the medical assistant's role in emergency care
- List the equipment and supplies maintained for emergencies in a medical office
- Explain the principles of early interventions with CPR and AED
- Discuss the types of emergencies that may be found in the medical offices and the appropriate interventions
- Define the role of the medical assistant in the GI medical office
- Describe the anatomy and physiology of the gastrointestinal system and accessory organs
- Discuss basic nutrition concepts
- Describe common diseases and disorders of the gastrointestinal system
- Describe common diagnostic procedures, treatments, and therapeutic diets for GI patients.

Lab Skills Discussion: *You will discuss the following hands-on skills in lab:*

- Procedure #23-1: Perform Adult Rescue Breathing and One-Rescuer CPR
- Procedure #23-2: Use an Automated External Defibrillator (AED)
- Procedure #23-3: Respond to an Adult with an Obstructed Airway
- Procedure #23-4: Administer Oxygen
- Procedure #23-5: Demonstrate the Application of a Pressure Bandage
- Procedure #23-7: Demonstrate the Application of a Splint
- Procedure #24-1: Assist with a Colon Endoscopic/Colonoscopy Exam
- Procedure #24-2: Assist with a Signoidoscopy
- Procedure #24-3: Insert a Rectal Suppository

Hands-On Lab Skill: *You will complete hands-on instruction in the following labs:*

- Procedure #23-6: Demonstrate a Triangular Sling

Student Slides: Slides E 42–46

Lesson Topics: *This lesson covers the following topics.*

- Emergency Resources
- Medical Office Preparedness
- Emergency Intervention
- The Anatomy and Physiology of the Gastrointestinal System
- Diseases and Disorders of the GI Tract
- Nutrition
- Diagnosis and Treatment of GI Disorders

Homework: *Complete the following assignments:*

- Read Chapters #25 and #26.
- Complete Chapter Reviews from Chapters #23 (pp. 497–498) and #24 (pp. 527–528).

LESSON #12: ORTHOPEDICS, PHYSICAL THERAPY, OBSTETRICS, AND GYNECOLOGY

Textbook:	*Clinical Medical Assisting: Foundations and Practices* by Frazier and Morgan
	Chapter #25: Orthopedics and Physical Therapy, pp. 529–562
	Chapter #26: Obstetrics and Gynecology, pp. 563–588
Objectives:	*After completing this lesson, you should be able to:*

- Describe the role of the medical assistant in the orthopedic office
- Describe the anatomy and physiology of the musculoskeletal system
- Discuss the diseases and disorders of the musculoskeletal system
- Discuss the diagnostic procedures and treatment modalities for musculoskeletal conditions
- Discuss the medical assistant's role in the obstetric/gynecology medical office
- Discuss the anatomy and physiology of the male and female reproductive system
- Discuss the disorders and conditions of the male and female reproductive systems
- Discuss the diagnostic tests, procedures, and treatments for reproductive disorders

Lab Skills Discussion: *You will complete hands-on instruction in the following labs:*
- Procedure #25-1: Assist with Fiberglass Cast Application
- Procedure #25-2: Assist with Cast Removal
- Procedure #25-3: Assist the Patient with Cold Application/Cold Compress
- Procedure #25-4: Assist the Patient with Hot Most Application/Hot Compress
- Procedure #25-5: Assist with Therapeutic Ultrasonography
- Procedure #25-6: Demonstrate Measuring for Axillary Crutches
- Procedure #25-7: Assist a Patient with Crutch Walking
- Procedure #25-8: Assist a Patient in Using a Cane
- Procedure #25-9: Assist a Patient in Using a Walker
- Procedure #25-10: Assist a Patient in a Wheelchair to and from an Exam Table
- Procedure #26-1: Assist with a Prenatal Exam
- Procedure #26-2: Instruct the Patient in Breast Self Examination
- Procedure #26-3: Assist in the Performance of a Pelvic Examination & Pap Test
- Procedure #26-4: Perform a Urine Pregnancy Test
- Procedure #26-5: Assist with Cryosurgery

Student Slides: Slides E 47-49

Quiz/Test (Start of class): Clinical Medical Assistant Quiz #2: Chapters 10, 11, 16, 18, 19, 20, 21, 22, 23, and 24

Lesson Topics: *This lesson covers the following topics.*
- The Anatomy and Physiology of the Musculoskeletal System
- Diseases, Disorders, and Treatment of Musculoskeletal Conditions in the Orthopedic Office
- The Anatomy and Physiology of the Reproductive Systems
- The Menstrual Cycle
- Contraception, Pregnancy, and Birth
- Gynecological Diseases and Disorders, Assessments, and Procedures

Homework: *Complete the following assignments:*
- Read Chapters #27 and #28.
- Complete Chapter Reviews from Chapters #25 (p. 561) and #26 (p. 587).

LESSON #13: PEDIATRICS AND NEUROLOGY

Textbook:
Clinical Medical Assisting: Foundations and Practices by Frazier and Morgan
Chapter #27: Pediatrics, pp. 589–608
Chapter #28: Neurology, pp. 609–626

Objectives:
After completing this lesson, you should be able to:

- Define the medical assistant's role in a pediatric specialty office
- Discuss the developmental factors relating to age of a child
- List the procedures that are performed during a well-child visit
- Discuss immunizations for children
- Discuss common diseases and disorders of children
- Discuss the diagnostic procedures used in a pediatric office
- Discuss the medical assistant's role in the neurology/neurosurgery practice
- Discuss the anatomy and physiology of the nervous system
- Discuss the various methods of neurological assessment
- Describe common diseases and disorders of the nervous system

Lab Skills Discussion:
You will discuss the following hands-on skills in lab:

- Procedure #27-1: Perform and Record Measurements of Height and Length, Weight, and head and Chest Circumference
- Procedure #27-2: Perform and Record Pediatric Vital Signs and Vision Screening
- Procedure #27-3: Perform Documentation of Immunizations, Both Stored and Administered
- Procedure #27-4: Perform Urine Collection with a Pediatric Urine Collection Bag
- Procedure #28-1: Assist in a Neurological Exam
- Procedure #28-2: Assist with a Lumbar Puncture
- Procedure #28-3: Prepare a patient for an Electroencephalogram

Student Slides:
Slides E 50–51

Lesson Topics:
This lesson covers the following topics.

- Physical, Developmental, and Emotional Growth of a Child
- Routine Visits
- Common Pediatric Diseases and Conditions
- Diagnostic Procedures
- The Anatomy and Physiology of the Nervous System
- Assessing the Neurological System
- Disorders and Diseases of the Nervous System
- Diseases of the Peripheral Nervous System

Homework:
Complete the following assignments:

- Read Chapters #29, #30, #31, and #32.
- Complete Chapter Reviews from Chapters #27 (pp. 607-608) and #28 (p. 625).

LESSON #14: MENTAL HEALTH, ONCOLOGY, GERIATRICS, AND ALTERNATIVE MEDICINE

Textbook:

Clinical Medical Assisting: Foundations and Practices by Frazier and Morgan
Chapter #29: Mental Health, pp. 627–643
Chapter #30: Oncology, pp. 644–654
Chapter #31: Geriatrics, pp. 655–665
Chapter #32: Alternative Medicine, pp. 668–678

Objectives:

After completing this lesson, you should be able to:
- Identify the medical assistant's role in the mental health field
- Describe selected psychological disorders and common assessments and treatments
- Identify the medical assistant's role in the oncology office
- Describe different types of malignant neoplasms including the staging and grading of malignancies
- Describe routine cancer screening and other diagnostic tests for cancer
- Discuss various treatments for cancer
- Explain the medical assistant's role in the geriatric medical office
- Discuss the physical, psychological, and social changes and factors related to aging
- Discuss the nutritional needs and challenges of the aging patient
- Describe measures to promote health in geriatric patients
- Describe selected types of alternative medicines

Lab Skills Discussion:

You will discuss the following hands-on skills in lab:
- Procedure #31-1: Role-Play Sensorimotor Changes of the Elderly

Student Slides:

Slides E 52–58

Lesson Topics:

This lesson covers the following topics.
- The Anatomy and Physiology of Cognitive Functioning
- Mental Wellness and Disorders
- Standard Treatments for Mental Disorders
- The Classification and physiology of Cancers
- Diagnostic Procedures
- Cancer Treatment
- Hospice and Emotional Support
- The Cancer Prevention Lifestyle
- The Aging Process
- Cultural Views of Aging
- Promoting Health Among the Elderly
- Complementary and Alternative Medical Systems
- Alternative Medicine
- Biologically Based Therapies
- Manipulative and Body-Based Methods
- Energy Therapies

Homework:

Complete the following assignments:
- Complete Chapter Reviews from Chapters #29 (pp. 642–643), #30 (pp. 653–654), #31 (p. 664), and #32 (p. 676)
- Read Chapters #1 and #2 in *EKG Technical Program Standard, Custom Edition*

Clinical Medical Assistant

EKG Technician Section Lesson Plans
Lessons #15–23

LESSON #15: CORONARY ANATOMY AND PHYSIOLOGY AND ELECTROPHYSIOLOGY

Textbook:	*EKG Technical Program Standard, Custom Edition* by Karen Ellis Chapter #1: Coronary Anatomy and Physiology, pp. 1–12 Chapter #2: Electrophysiology, pp. 13–33
Objectives:	*After completing this lesson, you should be able to:*

- Explain the anatomy and physiology of the cardiovascular system and related nervous control
- Explain the cardiac cycle
- Describe the *fight-or-flight* and *rest-and-digest* responses
- Explain the physiology of the electrical system of the heart
- Describe the waves of the EKG tracing
- Differentiate between the pacemakers of the heart and state the inherent rate of each
- Differentiate between *escape* and *usurpation*
- Identify selected arrhythmias

Handout:	Handout #1: Anatomy and Physiology of the Cardiovascular System Handout #2: The Conduction System
Student Slides:	Slides D 2–14
Quiz/Test (Start of class):	Clinical Medical Assistant Quiz #3: Chapters 25, 26, 27, 28, 29, 30, 31, and 32 in *Clinical Medical Assisting: Foundations and Practices* text
Lesson Topics:	*This lesson covers the following topics.*

- The Heart: Layers, Chambers, Valves, and Great Vessels
- Blood Flow through the Heart
- The Cardiac Cycle
- Diastole
- Systole
- Blood Flow through the Systemic Circulation
- Coronary Arteries
- Heart Cells

- Nervous Control of the Heart
- Depolarization and Repolarization
- The Action Potential and Refractory Periods
- EKG Waves and Complexes
- The Cardiac Conduction System
- Inherent Rates of the Pacemaker Cells
- Conduction Variations
- EKG Paper
- Intervals

Homework:	*Complete the following assignments:*

- Read Chapters #3 and #4.

LESSON #16: LEAD MORPHOLOGY AND PLACEMENT/TECHNICAL ASPECTS OF THE EKG

Textbook:	*EKG Technical Program Standard, Custom Edition* by Karen Ellis
	Chapter #3: Lead Morphology and Placement, pp. 35–46
	Chapter #4: Technical Aspects of the EKG, pp. 47–59
Objectives:	*After completing this lesson, you should be able to:*

- Define electrode
- Identify the bipolar leads and unipolar augmented leads
- Explain augmentation as it relates to the EKG
- Explain Einthoven's law and draw Einthoven's triangle
- Identify the leads composing the hexiaxial diagram
- Identify the precordial leads
- Describe the normal QRS complex deflections in each of the 12 leads of an EKG
- Explain the control features of an EKG machine
- Describe the different kinds of artifacts on a rhythm strip and explain how to troubleshoot each
- Differentiate between an artifact and a rhythm

Handout:	Handout #3: EKG Lead Placement
	Handout #4: The Blood Pressure, EKG Tracing, and Waves
	Handout #5: Patient Preparation and Safety
Student Slides:	Slides D 15–30
Hands-On Lab Skills:	*You will complete hands-on instruction in the following labs:*

- Introduction to the EKG Machine
- Patient Preparation and Safety
- 12-Lead Placement
- Performing a 12-Lead EKG
- Obtaining a Blood Pressure

Lesson Topics:	*This lesson covers the following topics.*

- Leads
- Continuous Monitoring
- Electrocardiographic Truths
- Normal QRS Deflections
- The EKG Machine
- Electrical Safety
- Artifacts
- Troubleshooting Artifacts
- Telemetry Monitoring

Homework:	*Complete the following assignments:*

- Read Chapters #5 and #6.

LESSON #17: CALCULATING HEART RATE AND RHYTHM STRIP INTERPRETATION

Textbook:

EKG Technical Program Standard, Custom Edition by Karen Ellis

Chapter #5: Calculating Heart Rate, pp. 61–72

Chapter #6: How to Interpret a Rhythm Strip, pp. 73–77

Objectives:

After completing this lesson, you should be able to:

- Define heart rate and calculate the heart rate on a variety of strips and using different methods
- Differentiate between the three types of rhythm regularity
- Identify the kind of heart rate to calculate for different kinds of rhythm regularity
- Use the five steps to interpret a variety of rhythms

Student Slides: Slides D 31–37

Quiz/Test (Start of class):   EKG Quiz #1: Chapters 1, 2, 3, and 4

Lesson Topics:

This lesson covers the following topics.

- Methods for Calculating Heart Rate
- Types of Regularity
- Calculating Heart Rate for Different Types of Regularity
- The Five Steps to Rhythm Interpretation

Homework:

Complete the following assignments:

- Read Chapter #7.

LESSON #18: RHYTHMS ORIGINATING IN THE SINUS NODE

Textbook:	*EKG Technical Program Standard, Custom Edition* by Karen Ellis
	Chapter #7: Rhythms Originating in the Sinus Node, pp. 79–98
Objectives:	*After completing this lesson, you should be able to:*

- State the criteria for each of the sinus rhythms
- Using the five steps, correctly interpret a variety of sinus rhythms on single- and double-lead strips
- State the adverse effects for each of the sinus rhythms
- State the possible treatment for the sinus rhythms

Handout:	Handout #6: Arrhythmias
	Handout #6A: Arrhythmia Chart
Hands-On Lab Skills:	*You will complete hands-on instruction in the following labs:*

- Performing a 12-Lead EKG

Student Slides:	Slides D 38–43
Lesson Topics:	*This lesson covers the following topics.*

- Sinus Rhythms
- Sinus Bradycardia
- Sinus Arrhythmia
- Sinus Arrest
- Sinus Block

Homework:	*Complete the following assignments:*

- Read Chapters #8 and #9.

LESSON #19: RHYTHMS ORIGINATING IN THE ATRIA AND AV JUNCTION

Textbook:	*EKG Technical Program Standard, Custom Edition* by Karen Ellis
	Chapter #8: Rhythms Originating in the Atria, pp. 99–119
	Chapter #9: Rhythms Originating in the AV Junction, pp. 121–132
Objectives:	*After completing this lesson, you should be able to:*

- State the criteria for each junctional rhythm
- Using the criteria and other rhythm analysis tools, correctly interpret a variety of atrial rhythms
- State the adverse effects and possible treatment for each rhythm
- State the criteria for each junctional rhythm
- Correctly identify the junctional rhythms using the criteria and the rhythm strip analysis tools
- State the adverse effects and possible treatments for each junctional rhythm.

Hands-On Lab Skills:	*You will complete hands-on instruction in the following labs:*

- Performing a 12-Lead EKG

Student Slides:	Slides D 44–53
Lesson Topics:	*This lesson covers the following topics.*

- Atrial Rhythms
- Wandering Atrial Pacemaker
- Premature Atrial Complexes
- Paroxysmal Atrial Tachycardia
- Atrial Flutter
- Atrial Fibrillation
- Supraventricular Tachycardia
- Junctional Rhythms
- Premature Junctional Complexes
- Junctional Bradycardia
- Junctional Rhythm
- Accelerated Junctional Rhythm
- Junctional Tachycardia

Homework:	*Complete the following assignments:*

- Read Chapter #10.

LESSON #20: RHYTHMS ORIGINATING IN THE VENTRICLES AND AV BLOCKS

Textbook:
EKG Technical Program Standard, Custom Edition by Karen Ellis

Chapter #10: Rhythms Originating in the Ventricles, pp. 133–155

Chapter #11: AV Blocks, pp. 157–176

Objectives:
After completing this lesson, you should be able to:

- State the criteria for each of the ventricular rhythms
- Correctly identify ventricular rhythms on a variety of strips
- State the adverse effects and possible treatment for the ventricular rhythms
- State the criteria for each type of AV block
- Identify each type of AV block
- State the adverse effects and possible treatment for each type of AV block

Hands-On Lab Skills:
You will complete hands-on instruction in the following labs:

- Performing a 12-Lead EKG

Student Slides:
Slides D 54–68

Quiz/Test (Start of class):
EKG Quiz #2: Chapters 5, 6, 7, 8, and 9

Lesson Topics:
This lesson covers the following topics.

- Ventricular Rhythms
- Premature Ventricular Complexes
- Agonal Rhythm
- Idioventricular Rhythm
- Accelerated Idioventricular Rhythm
- Ventricular Tachycardia and Fibrillation
- Torsades de Pointes
- Asystole
- Pacemakers
- Degrees of AV Blocks
- First Degree AV Block
- Type 1 Second-Degree AV Block (Wenckebach)
- Type II Second-Degree AV Block
- 2:1 AV Block
- Third-Degree AV Block (Complete Heart Block)

Homework:
Complete the following assignments:

- Read Chapter #12.

LESSON #21: RHYTHM PRACTICE STRIPS

Textbook: *EKG Technical Program Standard, Custom Edition* by Karen Ellis
                             Chapter #12: Rhythm Practice, pp. 177–301

Objectives: *After completing this lesson, you should be able to:*
                             • Correctly identify rhythms

Hands-On Lab Skills: *You will complete hands-on instruction in the following labs:*
                             • Performing a 12-Lead EKG

Student Slides: Slides D 69–79

Lesson Topics: *This lesson covers the following topics.*
                             • Sinus Rhythms
                             • Atrial Rhythms
                             • Junctional Rhythms
                             • Ventricular Rhythms
                             • AV Blocks
                             • Rhythm Regularity

Homework: *Complete the following assignments:*
                             • Read Chapter #13.

LESSON #22: ARTIFICIAL PACEMAKERS

Textbook: *EKG Technical Program Standard, Custom Edition* by Karen Ellis
                             Chapter #13: Pediatrics, pp. 303–317

Objectives: *After completing this lesson, you should be able to:*
- Explain the primary function of a pacemaker
- Outline indications for a pacemaker
- Name the components of a permanent pacemaker
- Describe the types of temporary pacemakers
- Define the terms firing, capture, and sensing
- State what each letter of the pacemaker code means
- Identify pacemaker rhythms and malfunctions

Handout: Handout #7: Pacemakers
                             Handout #8: Holter Monitor

Hands-On Lab Skills: *You will complete hands-on instruction in the following labs:*
- Performing a 12-Lead EKG

Student Slides: Slides D 80–83

Quiz/Test (Start of class): EKG Quiz #3: Chapters 10, 11, and 12

Lesson Topics: *This lesson covers the following topics.*
- Indications for an Artificial Pacemaker
- Permanent versus Temporary Pacemakers
- Pacemaker Terminology
- Three-Letter Pacemaker Code
- VVI Pacemakers
- DDD Pacemakers
- Pacemaker Malfunctions

Homework: *Complete the following assignments:*
- Read Chapter #14.

LESSON #23: DIAGNOSTIC ELECTROCARDIOGRAPHY

Textbook: *EKG Technical Program Standard, Custom Edition* by Karen Ellis

Chapter #14: Diagnostic Electrocardiography, pp. 319–346

Objectives: *After completing this lesson, you should be able to:*

- State the goals of and indications for stress testing
- Define MET
- Describe the relative and absolute contraindications to stress testing
- Demonstrate how to calculate target heart rate
- Explain the procedures for a stress test and a pharmacologic stress test
- Explain the three most commonly used protocols for treadmill exercise testing
- Describe the reasons to terminate the test
- Describe normal signs and symptoms and EKG changes during the stress test
- Explain Bayes's theorem
- Describe the indications and contraindications for Holter monitoring
- Describe the artifacts associated with Holter monitoring
- Differentiate between event monitoring and Holter monitoring

Handout: Handout #9: Echocardiography

Handout #10: EKG Study Guide

Hands-On Lab Skills: *You will complete hands-on instruction in the following labs:*

- Performing a 12-Lead EKG

Student Slides: Slides D 84–93

Lesson Topics: *This lesson covers the following topics.*

- Stress Testing
- Reliability of Stress Tests
- Categories of Stress Tests
- Holter Monitoring
- Event Monitoring

Clinical Medical Assistant

Lab Services and Phlebotomy Technician Section
Lesson Plans
Lessons #24–40

LESSON #24: PHLEBOTOMY PRACTICE AND QUALITY ASSESSMENT

Textbook:	*Phlebotomy Handbook* by Garza and Becan-McBride
	Chapter #1: Phlebotomy Practice and Quality Assessment, pp. 1–38
	Appendix #1: NAACLS Phlebotomy Competencies and Matrix, pp. 546–549
Objectives:	*After completing this lesson, you should be able to:*

- Describe the role of phlebotomy in patient care
- List professional competencies for phlebotomists and key elements of a performance assessment
- Explain components of professionalism and desired character traits for phlebotomists
- Describe coping skills that are used for stress in the workplace
- Distinguish between quality improvement and quality control

Handout:	Handout #1: Phlebotomy Practice and Quality Assessment
Student Slides:	Slides D 2–9
Lesson Topics:	*This lesson covers the following topics.*

- Phlebotomy Practice and Definition
- The Clinical Laboratory and Specimen Collection Services
- Competencies, Certification, and Professionalism for Phlebotomists
- Quality Improvement and Assessment

Homework:	*Complete the following assignments:*

- Review and complete questions pp. 34–38.

LESSON #25: COMMUNICATION, COMPUTERIZATION, AND DOCUMENTATION

Textbook: *Phlebotomy Handbook* by Garza and Becan-McBride

Chapter #2: Communication, Computerization, and Documentation, pp. 39–80

Appendix #4: Computer Basics, pp. 556–558

Objectives: *After completing this lesson, you should be able to:*

- Outline the basic communication loop
- Describe methods for effective verbal and nonverbal communication, active listening, and written communication
- Describe basic components of the medical record
- Explain how to maintain confidentiality and privacy of patient information
- Describe essential elements of laboratory test requisitions, specimen labels, and test results
- Identify essential components, functions, and uses of computers in health care

Handout: Handout #2: Communication, Computerization, and Documentation

Lab Skills Discussion: *You will complete hands-on instruction in the following labs:*

- Procedure 2-1: Initial Communication with the Deaf and/or Blind Patient

Student Slides: Slides D 10–14

Lesson Topics: *This lesson covers the following topics.*

- Communication Strategies for Health Care Workers
- Computer and Documentation basics
- Laboratory Test Requisitions, Specimen Labels, and Blood Collection Lists
- Specimen Labels
- Reporting Laboratory Results
- Documentation Essentials and the Medical Record

Homework: *Complete the following assignments:*

- Review and complete questions pp. 74–80.

LESSON #26: PROFESSIONAL ETHICS, LEGAL AND REGULATORY ISSUES, AND INFECTION CONTROL

Textbook:

Phlebotomy Handbook by Garza and Becan-McBride
Chapter #3: Professional Ethics, Legal, and Regulatory Issues, pp. 81–100
Chapter #4: Infection Control, pp. 101–137

Objectives:

After completing this lesson, you should be able to:
- Describe types of consent used in health care settings
- Describe how to avoid litigation as it relates to blood collection
- Define standard of care from a legal and a health care provider's perspective
- Explain HIPAA
- Explain the infection control policies and procedures that must be followed in specimen collection and transportation
- Identify basic programs for infection control and isolation procedures
- Explain proper techniques for handwashing, gowning, gloving, masking, double bagging, and entering and exiting isolation areas
- Identify steps to avoid transmission of blood-borne pathogens
- Identify ways to reduce risks for accidental needlesticks
- Identify the steps to take in the case of blood-borne pathogen exposure

Handout:

Handout #3: Professional Ethics, Legal, and Regulatory Issues
Handout #4: Infection Control

Lab Skills Discussion:

You will complete hands-on instruction in the following labs:
- Procedure 4-1: Handwashing Technique
- Procedure 4-5: Disposing of Contaminated Items
- Procedure 4-6: Removal of Patient's Specimen from Isolation Room

Hands-On Lab Skills:

You will discuss the following hands-on skills in lab:
- Procedure 4-2: Donning and Removing Gloves
- Procedure 4-3: Gowning, Masking, and Gloving
- Procedure 4-4: Removal Isolation Gown, Mask, and Gloves

Student Slides:

Slides D 15–24

Lesson Topics:

This lesson covers the following topics.
- Ethics
- Patients' Rights
- Governmental Laws
- Basic Legal Principles
- Legal Claims and Defense
- HIV-Related Issues
- Professional Liability Insurance
- Pathogens and Infections
- Personal Safety from Infection During Specimen Handling
- Chain of Infection
- Standard precautions
- Specific isolation Techniques and Procedural Steps
- Infection Control and Safety in the Clinical Laboratory

Homework:

Complete the following assignments:
- Review and complete questions pp. 97–100 and 134–137.

LESSON #27: SAFETY AND FIRST AID, MEDICAL TERMINOLOGY, AND ANATOMY AND PHYSIOLOGY OF ORGAN SYSTEMS

Textbook:
Phlebotomy Handbook by Garza and Becan-McBride
Chapter #5: Safety and First Aid, pp. 138–157
Chapter #6: Medical Terminology, Anatomy and Physiology of Organ Systems, pp. 158–206

Objectives:
After completing this lesson, you should be able to:
- Explain the measures that should be taken for fire, electrical, radiation, mechanical, and chemical safety in a health care facility
- Describe the essential elements of a disaster emergency plan for a health care facility
- Explain the safety policies and procedures that must be followed in specimen collection and transportation
- describe the safe use of equipment in healthcare facilities
- List three precautions that can reduce the risk of injury to patients
- Describe how laboratory testing is used to assess body functions and disease
- Describe the directional terms, anatomic surface regions, and cavities of the body
- Describe homeostasis
- Describe the purpose, function, and structural components of the major body systems
- Identify examples of pathologic conditions and diagnostic tests associated with each organ system
- Describe the types of specimens that are analyzed in the clinical laboratory

Handout:
Handout #5: Safety and First Aid
Handout #6: Med Term, Anatomy and Physiology of Organ Systems

Lab Skills Discussion:
You will discuss the following hands-on skills in lab:
- Procedures 5-1: Breathing Aid

Student Slides:
Slides D 25–48

Lesson Topics:
This lesson covers the following topics.
- Fire Safety
- Electrical Safety
- Radiation Safety
- Mechanical Safety
- Chemical Safety
- Equipment and Safety in Patients' Rooms
- Patient Safety Outside the Room
- Patient Safety Related to Latex Products
- Disaster Emergency Plan
- Emergency Procedures
- Medical Terminology
- Anatomy and Physiology Overview
- Anatomic Regions and Positions
- Major Organ Systems

Homework:
Complete the following assignments:
- Review and complete questions pp. 154–157 and 200–206.

LESSON #28: THE CARDIOVASCULAR AND LYMPHATIC SYSTEMS

Textbook: *Phlebotomy Handbook* by Garza and Becan-McBride

Chapter #7: The Cardiovascular and Lymphatic Systems, pp. 207–248

Objectives: *After completing this lesson, you should be able to:*

- Define the anatomy and physiology of the cardiovascular and lymphatic systems
- List pathologic conditions and common laboratory tests associated with the cardiovascular and lymphatic systems
- Describe the properties of arterial blood, venous blood, and capillary blood
- Describe the cellular and noncellular components of blood
- Differentiate between whole blood, serum, and plasma
- Locate and name the veins most commonly used for phlebotomy procedures
- Define hemostasis and explain the basic process of coagulation and fibrinolysis

Handout: Handout #7: The Cardiovascular and Lymphatic Systems

Student Slides: Slides D 49–62

Quiz: Phlebotomy Quiz #1: Chapters 1, 2, 3, 4, 5, and 6

Lesson Topics: *This lesson covers the following topics.*

- The Cardiovascular System
- The Heart
- The Vessels and Circulation
- The Blood
- Hemostasis and Coagulation
- Lymphatic System

Homework: *Complete the following assignments:*

- Review and complete questions pp. 244–248.

LESSON #29: BLOOD COLLECTION EQUIPMENT

Textbook: *Phlebotomy Handbook* by Garza and Becan-McBride

Chapter #8: Blood Collection Equipment, pp. 249–280

Objectives: *After completing this lesson, you should be able to:*

- Describe phlebotomy safety supplies and equipment
- List types of anticoagulants and additives used in blood collection, their mechanisms of action on collected blood, examples of tests performed on these tubes and their vacuum collection tube color codes
- Identify the supplies that should be carried on a specimen collection tray when collecting blood by venipuncture or skin puncture
- Identify the safety equipment needed to collect blood by venipuncture and skin puncture

Handout: Handout #8: Blood Collection Equipment

Student Slides: Slides D 63–70

Lesson Topics: *This lesson covers the following topics.*

- Venipuncture Equipment
- Blood Collection Tubes and Additives
- Safety Syringes
- Tourniquets
- Vensocope
- Bleeding-Time Equipment
- Gloves for Blood Collection
- Antiseptics, Sterile Gauze Pads, and bandages
- Microcollection Equipment
- Blood-Drawing Chair
- Infant Phlebotomy Station
- Specimen Collection Trays

Homework: *Complete the following assignments:*

- Review and complete questions pp. 277–280.

LESSON #30: PREANALYTICAL COMPLICATIONS CAUSING MEDICAL ERRORS IN BLOOD COLLECTION

Textbook:

Phlebotomy Handbook by Garza and Becan-McBride

Chapter #9: Preanalytical Complications Causing Medical Errors in Blood Collection, pp. 281–300

Objectives:

After completing this lesson, you should be able to:

- Describe preanalytical complications related to phlebotomy procedures
- Explain how to prevent and/or handle complications in blood collection
- List factors that can affect blood collection
- List preanalytical complications that can arise with test requests and identification
- Describe complications associated with tourniquet pressure and fist pumping
- Describe methods used to prevent preanalytical complications in blood collection

Handout:

Handout #9: Preanalytical Complications Causing Medical Errors in Blood Collection

Student Slides:

Slides D 71–80

Lesson Topics:

This lesson covers the following topics.

- Categories of Preanalytical Variables
- Complications Associated with Test Requests and Identification
- Complications Associated with the Specimen Collection Procedure

Homework:

Complete the following assignments:

- Review and complete questions pp. 297–300.

LESSON #31: VENIPUNCTURE PROCEDURES

Textbook:	*Phlebotomy Handbook* by Garza and Becan-McBride
	Chapter #10: Venipuncture Procedures, pp. 301–362
Objectives:	*After completing this lesson, you should be able to:*

- Describe the steps in preparing for a venipuncture procedures
- List the supplies and equipment used in a venipuncture procedure
- Describe the steps in patient identification process and what to do if information is missing
- Describe the methods for hand hygiene
- Identify the appropriate sites for venipuncture and situations when these sites might not be acceptable as well as alternative sites
- Describe the process for applying a tourniquet to a patient's arm
- Describe the decontamination process and agents used to decontaminate skin for routine blood tests and blood cultures
- Describe the steps for of a venipuncture procedure using the evacuated tube method, syringe method, and butterfly method according to the CLSI Approved Standard

Handout:	Handout #10: Venipuncture Procedures
Hands-On Lab Skills:	*You will complete hands-on instruction in the following labs:*

- Procedure 10-1: Preparing for the Patient Encounter
- Procedure 10-2: Hand Hygiene and Gloving Technique
- Procedure 10-3: Basics of Patient Identification
- Procedure 10-4: Use of a Tourniquet and Vein Palpation
- Procedure 10-5: Decontamination of the Puncture Site
- Procedure 10-6: Performing a Venipuncture
- Procedure 10-7: Syringe Method

Student Slides:	Slides D 81–105
Lesson Topics:	*This lesson covers the following topics.*

- Blood Collection
- Health Care Worker Preparation
- Needlestick prevention Strategies
- Approaching, Assessing, and Identifying the Patient
- Equipment Selection and Preparation
- Venipuncture Methods

Homework:	*Complete the following assignments:*

- Review and complete questions pp. 356–362.

LESSON #32: CAPILLARY BLOOD SPECIMENS

Textbook: *Phlebotomy Handbook* by Garza and Becan-McBride
                        Chapter #11: Capillary Blood Specimens, pp. 363–382

Objectives: *After completing this lesson, you should be able to:*

- Describe the reasons for acquiring capillary blood specimens
- List the laboratory tests for which capillary specimens may be collected
- Identify the proper sites for performing a skin puncture procedure
- Describe the procedure for performing a skin puncture
- Describe the procedure for making blood smears

Handout: Handout #11: Capillary Blood Specimens

Hands-On Lab Skills: *You will complete hands-on instruction in the following labs:*

- Procedure 11-1: Acquiring a Capillary Blood Specimen (Skin Puncture) using a Retractable Safety Device
- Procedure 11-2: Blood Smears/Films for Microscopic Slides

Student Slides: Slides D 106–115

Lesson Topics: *This lesson covers the following topics.*

- Indications for Skin Puncture
- Composition of Capillary Blood
- Basic Technique for Collecting Diagnostic Capillary Blood Specimens
- Preparation for Skin Puncture
- Supplies for Skin Puncture
- Skin Puncture Sites
- Skin Puncture Procedure
- Order of Collection
- Blood Films for Microscopic Slides
- Other Considerations for Capillary Blood Samples
- Lancet Disposal, Labeling the Specimen, and Completing the Interaction

Homework: *Complete the following assignments:*

- Review and complete questions pp. 379–382.

LESSON #33: SPECIMEN HANDLING, TRANSPORTATION, AND PROCESSING

Textbook:	*Phlebotomy Handbook* by Garza and Becan-McBride
	Chapter #12: Specimen Handling, Transportation, and Processing, pp. 383–404
Objectives:	*After completing this lesson, you should be able to:*
	• Describe sources of preexamination error that can occur during blood specimen handling, transportation, processing, and storage
	• Describe methods commonly used to transport specimens
Handout:	Handout #12: Specimen Handling, Transportation, and Processing
Hands-On Lab Skills:	*You will complete hands-on instruction in the following labs:*
	• Hands-on Venipuncture Practice
Student Slides:	Slides D 116–125
Lesson Topics:	*This lesson covers the following topics.*
	• Specimen Handling After the Venipuncture
	• Specimen Delivery Methods
	• Processing the Specimen on Arrival at the Clinical Laboratory
	• Reporting Laboratory Results
Homework:	*Complete the following assignments:*
	• Review and complete questions pp. 400–404.

LESSON #34: PEDIATRIC AND GERIATRIC PROCEDURES

Textbook: *Phlebotomy Handbook* by Garza and Becan-McBride

                       Chapter #13: Pediatric and Geriatric Procedures, pp. 405–443

Objectives: *After completing this lesson, you should be able to:*

- Describe the fears that children in different developmental stages might have toward the blood collection process and ways that these fears can be handled
- Describe puncture sites and the procedures for a heel stick on an infant
- Describe the venipuncture sites, equipment and supplies, and procedures for infants and young children
- Explain the special precautions and types of equipment needed to collect capillary blood gases
- Describe the procedure for specimen collection for neonatal screening
- Define physical and/or emotional changes that are associated with the aging process and appropriate responses to these changes by healthcare workers

Handout: Handout #13: Pediatric and Geriatric Procedures

Lab Skills Discussion: *You will discuss the following hands-on skills in lab:*

- Procedure 13-1: Heel Stick Procedure
- Procedure 13-2: Collection for Capillary Blood Gas Testing
- Procedure 13-3: Collection of Capillary Blood for Neonatal Screening
- Procedure 13-4: Procedure for Heparin or Saline Lock Blood Collection
- Procedure 13-5: Procedure for Central Venous Catheter Blood Collection

Hands-On Lab Skills: *You will complete hands-on instruction in the following labs:*

- Hands-on Venipuncture Practice

Student Slides: Slides D 126–141

Quiz: Phlebotomy Quiz #2: Chapters 7, 8, 9, 10, 11, and 12

Lesson Topics: *This lesson covers the following topics.*

- Pediatric Patients
- Age-Specific Care Considerations
- Preparing Child and Parent
- Positions for Restraining a Child
- Combative Patients
- Decreasing the Needlestick Pain
- Precautions to Protect the Child
- Latex Allergy Alert
- Pediatric Phlebotomy Procedures
- Geriatric Patients

Homework: *Complete the following assignments:*

- Review and complete questions pp. 440–443.

LESSON #35: POINT-OF-CARE COLLECTIONS

Textbook: *Phlebotomy Handbook* by Garza and Becan-McBride

Chapter #14: Point-of-Care Collections, pp. 444–464

Objectives: *After completing this lesson, you should be able to:*

- Identify analytes whose levels can be determined through point-of-care testing
- Define quality assurance and its requirements in point-of-care testing
- Describe the equipment that is used to perform the bleeding-time test

Handout: Handout #14: Point of Care Collections

Lab Skills Discussion: *You will discuss the following hands-on skills:*

- Procedure 14-1: Obtaining Blood Specimen for Glucose Testing (Skin Puncture)
- Procedure 14-2: Surgicutt Bleeding-Time Test

Hands-On Lab Skills: *You will complete hands-on instruction in the following labs:*

- Hands-on Venipuncture Practice

Student Slides: Slides D 142–154

Lesson Topics: *This lesson covers the following topics.*

- Glucose Monitoring
- Blood Gas and Electrolyte Analysis
- Point-of-Care Testing for Acute Heart Damage
- Blood Coagulation Monitoring
- Hematocrit, Hemoglobin, and Other Hematology Parameters
- Cholesterol Screening
- Bleeding-Time Test
- Other POCT Tests

Homework: *Complete the following assignments:*

- Review and complete questions pp. 461–464.

LESSON #36: ARTERIAL, INTRAVENOUS, AND SPECIAL COLLECTION PROCEDURES

Textbook:	*Phlebotomy Handbook* by Garza and Becan-McBride
	Chapter #15: Arterial, Intravenous (IV), and Special Collection Procedures, pp. 465–499
Objectives:	*After completing this lesson, you should be able to:*

- Explain the steps and equipment in blood culture collections
- Discuss the requirements for the glucose and lactose tolerance test
- Differentiate cannulas from fistulas
- List the special requirements for collecting blood through intravenous catheters
- Differentiate therapeutic phlebotomy from autologous transfusion
- Describe the special precautions needed to collect blood in therapeutic drug monitoring procedures
- List the types of patient specimens that are needed for trace metal analyses

Handout:	Handout #15: Arterial, Intravenous (IV), and Special Collection Procedures
Lab Skills Discussion:	*You will discuss the following hands-on skills in lab:*

- Procedure 15-2: Safety Syringe Blood Culture Collection
- Procedure 15-7: Collecting Blood Through a CVC

Hands-On Lab Skills:	*You will complete hands-on instruction in the following labs:*

- Procedure 15-1: Site-Preparation for Blood Culture Collection
- Procedure 15-3: Safety Butterfly Assembly Blood Culture Collection
- Procedure 15-4: Evacuated Tube System for Blood Culture Collection
- Procedure 15-5: After Blood Culture Collection by the Previous Methods
- Procedure 15-6: Radial ABG Procedure

Student Slides:	Slides D 155–170
Lesson Topics:	*This lesson covers the following topics.*

- Blood Cultures
- Glucose Tolerance Test (GTT)
- Postprandial Glucose Test
- Modified Oral Glucose Tolerance Test
- Lactose Tolerance Test
- Arterial Blood Gases
- Therapeutic Drug Monitoring (TDM)
- Collection for Trace Metals (Elements)
- Genetic Molecular Tests
- IV Line Collections
- Cannulas and Fistulas
- Donor Room Collections
- Autologous Transfusion
- Therapeutic Phlebotomy

Homework:	*Complete the following assignments:*

- Review and complete questions pp. 496–499.

LESSON #37: URINALYSIS, BODY FLUID, AND OTHER SPECIMENS

Textbook: *Phlebotomy Handbook* by Garza and Becan-McBride

Chapter #16: Urinalysis, Body Fluids, and Other Specimens, pp. 500–522

Objectives: *After completing this lesson, you should be able to:*

- Identify the body fluid specimens that are analyzed in the clinical laboratory and the correct procedures for collecting and transporting these specimens to the laboratory
- Describe the correct methodology for labeling urine specimens
- Instruct a patient on the correct procedure for collecting a timed urine specimen and a midstream clean-catch specimen

Handout: Handout #16: Urinalysis, Body Fluid, and Other Specimens

Lab Skills Discussion: *You will complete hands-on instruction in the following labs:*

- Procedure 16-1: Clean-Catch Midstream Urine Collection Instructions for Women
- Procedure 16-2: Clean-Catch Midstream Urine Collection Instructions for Men
- Procedure 16-3: Collecting a 24-Hour Urine Specimen
- Procedure 16-4: Collecting a Sputum Specimen
- Procedure 16-5: Collecting a Throat Swab for Culture

Hands-On Lab Skills: *You will complete hands-on instruction in the following labs:*

- Hands-on Venipuncture Practice

Student Slides: Slides D 171–180

Lesson Topics: *This lesson covers the following topics.*

- Urine Collection
- Cerebrospinal Fluid
- Fecal Specimens
- Seminal Fluid
- Amniotic Fluid
- Other Body Fluids
- Culture Specimens
- Sweat Chloride by Iontophoresis

Homework: *Complete the following assignments:*

- Review and complete questions pp. 519–522.

LESSON #38: DRUG USE, FORENSIC TOXICOLOGY, WORKPLACE TESTING, SPORTS MEDICINE, AND RELATED AREAS

Textbook:	*Phlebotomy Handbook* by Garza and Becan-McBride
	Chapter #17: Drug Use, Forensic Toxicology, Workplace Testing, Sports Medicine, and Related Areas, pp. 523–544
Objectives:	*After completing this lesson, you should be able to:*

- Describe specimens that can be used for forensic analysis
- Describe the role of the healthcare worker when working with forensic specimens
- Describe the role of the phlebotomist in federal drug-testing programs
- Describe the function of a chain of custody and the Custody and Control Form
- Describe how to detect adulteration of urine specimens
- Describe methods of measuring blood alcohol content
- Describe factors that affect testing for alcohol content

Handout:	Handout #17: Drug Use, Forensic Toxicology, Workplace Testing, Sports Medicine, and Related Areas
Hands-On Lab Skills:	*You will complete hands-on instruction in the following labs:*

- Hands-On Venipuncture Practice

Student Slides:	Slides D 181–186
Lesson Topics:	*This lesson covers the following topics.*

- Overview and Prevalence of Drug Use
- Common Drug Analysis Methods and Interferences
- Forensic Toxicology Specimens
- Chain of Custody
- Workplace Drug Testing
- Tampering with Specimens
- Drug Testing in the Private Sector
- Drug Use in Sports
- Preferred Specimens for Drug Tests
- Neonatal Drug Testing
- Blood Alcohol and Breath Testing

Homework:	*Complete the following assignments:*

- Review and complete questions pp. 541–544.

LESSON #39: FINDING A JOB AND THE BASICS OF VITAL SIGNS

Textbook: *Phlebotomy Handbook* by Garza and Becan-McBride

Appendix #2: Finding a Job, pp. 550–554

Appendix #5: The Basics of Vital Signs, pp. 559–569

Objectives: *After completing this lesson, you should be able to:*

- Describe strategies to find a job in the healthcare field
- Write an effective cover letter for sending to a potential employer
- Create an effective resume
- Respond appropriately to common interview questions
- Describe considerations to be used when deciding on accepting a job
- Explain the procedures for taking the following vital signs: temperature, pulse, blood pressure, respiration rate
- Describe how to report vital signs

Student Workbook: Certification Exam Review: NHA and CCMA Study Guide

Lab Skills Discussion: *You will discuss the following hands-on skills in lab:*

- Procedure A5-2: Taking Aural Temperature
- Procedure A5-3: Taking Axillary Temperature

Hands-On Lab Skills: *You will complete hands-on instruction in the following labs:*

- Procedure A5-1: Taking Oral Temperature
- Procedure A5-4: Assessing Peripheral Pulse Rate
- Procedure A5-5: Taking Blood Pressure
- Procedure A5-6: Assessing Respiration Rate

Student Slides: Slides D 187–197

Quiz: Phlebotomy Quiz #3: Chapters 13, 14, 15, 16, and 17

Lesson Topics: *This lesson covers the following topics.*

- Job Search Strategies
- The Cover Letter
- The Resume
- The Interview
- Decision Considerations
- Vital Signs

Homework: *Complete the following assignments:*

- Study for the Final Exam.

LESSON #40: CMA FINAL EXAM

Textbook: *Phlebotomy Handbook* by Garza and Becan-McBride

                                       N/A

Student Workbook: Certification Exam Review NHA-CCMA Study Guide

Final Exam: CMA Final Exam

PART B
Clinical Medical Assistant

STUDENT HANDOUTS

TABLE OF CONTENTS

Page

Handout #1   What Is HIPPA? B-3

Handout #1a   Study Notes for Medical Terminology (Separate Attachment) B-7

Handout #2   Common Abbreviations B-9

Handout #3   Patient History Form B-15

Handout #4   Medical Records B-19

Handout #5   Body Mechanics B-23

Handout #6   Peripheral Intravenous B-29

Handout #7   NHA CCMA Certification Review Guide (Separate Attachment) B-47

The Clinical Medical Assistant Program

Handout #1

WHAT IS HIPAA?

WHAT IS HIPAA?

The Health Insurance Portability and Accountability Act of 1996 (HIPAA) consists of two Titles. Title I protects health insurance coverage for workers and their families when they change or lose their jobs. Title II requires the Department of Health and Human Services (HHS) to establish national standards for electronic health care transactions and addresses the security and privacy of health information.

WHAT IS THE PRIVACY RULE?

The Privacy Rule is a federal regulation defining administrative steps, policies, and procedures to safeguard individuals' personal, private health information (protected health information or PHI).

WHEN DOES THE PRIVACY RULE BECOME EFFECTIVE?

President Bush approved the regulations on April 12, 2001. The official effective date of the regulations is April 14, 2001. <u>Covered entities, including hospitals and physicians, have two (2) years to comply (by April 14, 2003)</u>, except for small health plans which have until April 14, 2004 to comply.

WHO MUST COMPLY WITH THE PRIVACY RULE?

The following types of health care organizations are defined as "covered entities" by the Privacy Rule:

- All health care providers who choose to transmit certain administrative and financial health information electronically.
- All health plans.

- All health care clearinghouses

Covered entities may disclose health information to persons or organizations they hire to perform functions on their behalf (e.g. legal or accounting services). These "business associates" would not be permitted, under contractual obligation with the covered entity, to use or disclose protected health information in ways that would not be permitted of the covered entity itself.

WHAT INFORMATION IS PROTECTED?

The rule defines "protected health information" as health information that

1. identifies an individual and

2. is maintained or exchanged electronically or in hard copy.

If the information has any components that could be used to identify a person, it would be protected.

ARE THERE PENALTIES?

HIPAA calls for severe civil and criminal penalties for non-compliance, including:

- fines up to $25K for multiple violations of the same standard in a calendar year
- fines up to $250K and/or imprisonment up to 10 years for knowing misuse of individually identifiable health information

THE RULES UNDER HIPAA

1. Standards for Electronic Transactions
   The term **"Electronic Health Transactions"** includes health claims, health plan eligibility, enrollment and disenrollment, payments for care and health plan premiums, claim status, first injury reports, coordination of benefits, and related transactions.

2. Unique Identifiers for Providers, Employers, and Health Plans
   In the past, healthcare organizations have used multiple identification formats when conducting business with each other—a confusing, error-prone and costly approach. It is expected that standard identifiers will reduce these problems. The Employer Identifier Standard, published in 2002, adopts an employer's tax ID number or employer identification number (EIN) as the standard for electronic transactions.

3. Security Rule
   The final Security Rule was published on February 20, 2003 and provides for a uniform level of protection of all health information that is housed or transmitted electronically and that pertains to an individual. The Security Rule requires covered entities to ensure the confidentiality, integrity, and availability of all electronic protected health information (ePHI) the covered entity creates, receives, maintains, or transmits. It also requires entities to protect against any reasonably anticipated threats or hazards to the security or integrity of ePHI, protect against any reasonably anticipated uses or disclosures of such information that are not permitted or required by the Privacy Rule, and ensure compliance by their workforce.

4. Privacy Rule
   The Privacy Rule is intended to protect the privacy of all individually identifiable health information in the hands of covered entities, regardless of whether the information is or has been in

electronic form. Restrict most disclosures of protected health information to the minimum needed for healthcare treatment and business operations

- Provide that all patients are formally notified of covered entities' privacy practices,
- Enable patients to decide if they will authorize disclosure of their protected health information (PHI) for uses other than treatment or healthcare business operations
- Establish new criminal and civil sanctions for improper use or disclosure of PHI
- Implement a comprehensive compliance program, including
    - Conducting an impact assessment to determine gaps between existing information practices and policies and HIPAA requirements
    - Reviewing functions and activities of the organization's business partners to determine where Business Associate Agreements are required
    - Developing and implementing enterprise-wise privacy policies and procedures to implement the Rule
    - Assigning a Privacy officer who will administer the organizational privacy program and enforce compliance
    - Training all members of the workforce on HIPAA and organizational privacy policies
    - Updating systems to ensure they provide adequate protection of patient data

The Clinical Medical Assistant Program

Handout #1a

MEDICAL TERMINOLOGY STUDY NOTES

See Attachment:
Study Notes for Medical Terminology: Get Connected! by Suzanne S. Frucht
ISBN-10: 0132724251
ISBN-13: 9780132724258
Publisher: Prentice Hall
Copyright: 2012

The Clinical Medical Assistant Program

Handout #2

COMMON ABBREVIATIONS

A

ABG	
ABO	A system of classifying blood groups
a.c.	Before meals
ADL	Activities of daily living
AIDS	Acquired immunodeficiency syndrome
AP	Anterioposterior
A&P	Anterior and posterior, Anatomy & Physiology
ARDS	Adult respiratory distress syndrome *(most ill/sick pts.) ventilators*

B

bact	Bacteriology
bid	Twice a day *(every 12 Hours)*
BP	Blood pressure
bpm	Beats per minute
BSA	Body surface area — *Burn victims*
BUN	Blood urea nitrogen
BX,	Bx Biopsy

C

C	Celsius, centigrade, complement
c̄	With
Ca, ca	Cancer, carcinoma
CAG's, CAB	Coronary artery grafts, Coronary artery bypass
caps	Capsules

CCF	Congestive cardiac failure
CCU	Coronary care unit
cg	Centigram
CHF	Congestive heart failure
cm	Centimeter
CNS	Central nervous system
COPD	Chronic obstructive pulmonary disease
CPR	Cardiopulmonary resuscitation, C-reactive protein
C&S	Culture and sensitivity
CSF	Cerebrospinal fluid
CT, CAT	Computerized tomography, Computerized axial tomography
CVA	Cerebrovascular accident

D

D&C	Dilatation and curettage
D&V	Diarrhea and vomiting
DIC	Disseminated intravascular coagulation
DIFF, diff	Differential blood count
DM	Diabetes mellitus
DNA	Deoxyribonucleic acid
DOA	Dead on arrival
DPT	Diphtheria, pertussis, and tetanus (toxoids/vaccine)
DT's	Delirium tremens
D/W	Dextrose in water
Dx	Diagnosis

E

ECG	Electrocardiogram
ED	Emergency department
EEG	Electroencephalogram
ENT	Ear, nose, and throat
ESR	Erythrocyte sedimentation rate
exc	Excision

F

F	Fahrenheit
Fe	Iron
FBS, FBG	Fasting blood sugar/glucose
ft	Foot, feet (measure)
FUO	Fever of undetermined (unknown) origin

G

g, gm	Gram
GI	Gastrointestinal
GP	General practitioner
gr	Grain
gt, gtt	Drop, drops
GTT	Glucose tolerance test
GYN, gyn	Gynecology

H

Hb	Hemoglobin

HCG	Human chorionic gonadotropin
Hgb	Hemoglobin
HR	Heart rate
Hr	Hour
Hx	History

I

ICU	Intensive care unit
I.M.	Intramuscular
IN	Intra-nasal
In situ	In place
inf	Inferior
inj	Inject
I&O	Intake and output
IPPB	Intermittent positive-pressure breathing
IUD	Intrauterine device
IV	Intravenous

K

K	Potassium
kg	kilogram
KO	Keep open
KVO	Keep vein open

L

L, l	Liter
lat	lateral
lb	Pound
LBBB	Left bundle branch block
LFT	Liver function test
LH	Luteinizing hormone
LLL	Left lower lobe
LOC	Loss of conciousness
LOS	Length of stay
L/S	Lying/Standing
Lt, L)	left
LUQ	Left upper quadrant
LV	Left ventricle

M

m	Meter, minim
MD	Medical doctor, muscular dystrophy
MI	Myocardial infarction
MRSA	Methicillin resistant staphylococcus aureus
MSU	Midstream specimen of urine
MRI	Magnetic resonance imaging

N

Na	Sodium
NAD	No abnormalities detected
NIDDM	Non insulin dependant diabetes
NKA	No known allergies

| NPO | Nothing by mouth / Nil orally |
| NOAD | No other abnormalities detected |

O
O/A	On arrival
Ob-GYN	Obstetrics and gynaecology
OTC	Over the counter
oz	Ounce
O2	Oxygen
O2 Sat	Oxygen saturation levels

P
PAC	Pressure area care
Path	Pathology
Pap	Papanicolaou smear
PCA	Patient controlled analgesia
p.c.	After meals (post cibum)
peds	Pediatrics
Perrla, Pearl	Puplis equal, round, react to light and accommodation or Pupils equal & reacting to light
PHx	Past history
PID	Pelvic inflammatory disease
PMS	Premenstrual syndrome
PU	Passed urine
PUO	Pyrexia of unknown origen
PVC	Premature ventricular contraction
PV	per vagina

Q
q	Every
q.d.	Every day
q.h.	Every hour
q2h	Every 2 hours
q4h	Every 4 hours
q.i.d.	Four times a day

R
R	Respirations, roentgen
RA	Rheumatoid arthritis
RIB	Rest in bed
R/O	Rule out
ROM	Range of motion (of joint)
R/V	Review
Rx	Treatment

S
s*	Without
S.C., SQ, subq	Subcutaneous
sec	Second
sed rate	Sedimentation rate
SIDS	Sudden infant death syndrome
SOB	Short of breath

SOBOE	Short of breath on exertion
spec	Specimin
Sub Cut	Sub-cutaneous
Supps.	Suppository
S&S	Signs and symptoms
ss*	One-half
stat	Immediately
STD	Sexually transmitted disease
Sx	Symptoms
T	
T	Temperature (thoracic, to be followed by number designating specific thoracic vertebra EG T2)
T&A	Tonsillectomy and adenoidectomy
Tabs	Tablets
T&C	Type and cross-match
temp.	Temperature
THR	Total hip replacement
TIA	Transient ischemic attack
t.i.d.	Three times a day
TMJ	Temporomandibular joint
TPN	Total parenteral nutrition
TPR	Temperature, pulse, respirations
tsp	Teaspoon
U	
ung	Ointment
URI	Upper respiratory infection
UTI	Urinary tract infection
V	
VDRL	Venereal Disease Research Laboratory (test for syphilis)
VF	Ventricular fibrillation
VS	Vital signs
W	
WBC	White blood cell
WHO	World Health Organization
W/Walker	Wheelie walker
Wt	Weight

The Clinical Medical Assistant Program

Handout #3

PATIENT HISTORY FORM

(To be used to complete Procedure 6-2 in the Textbook)

Your Name: _____ Date of Birth: _____

Date you are filling out this form: _____

What type of complaint or disease is the reason for requesting this visit?

_____

TELL US ABOUT YOURSELF:
Home situation (circle, or add in writing):

Single _____ Married (how long _____) Divorced (how long _____) Widowed (how long _____)

Domestic partnership _____ Children? _____ Are they healthy? _____

Employment:

Status: full-time _____ part-time _____ retired _____ disabled _____ homemaker _____

Occupation/type of work/jobs: _____

Habits: Do you smoke? No _____ Yes _____ If yes, how many packs per day? _____

If you have quit, how long ago? _____

Do you use alcohol? No _____ Yes _____ If yes, how often do you drink? _____

If you have quit, how long ago? _____

Do family or friends worry about your alcohol intake? _____

Have you ever had problems with drug use? _____

PAST MEDICAL HISTORY:

Please list other diseases from which you <u>currently</u> suffer (heart, lung, etc.):

_____

_____

Please list other medical conditions from which you have suffered in the past:

_____

_____

Please list any surgeries (operations), reason for the surgery, and date of surgery:

_____

_____

MEDICATIONS:

Prescription medications	Dose	How often taken

NON-PRESCRIPTION (over-the-counter medications) such as aspirin, ibuprofen, vitamins, laxatives, etc.)

Over-the-counter medications	Dose	How often taken

HERBAL PREPARATIONS

Herbal preparation	Dose	How often taken

ALLERGIES OR ADVERSE DRUG REACTIONS? Please list drug and type of reaction:

_____

FAMILY HISTORY:
Place an "X" in appropriate boxes to identify all illnesses/conditions in your blood relatives.

Illness/Condition	Family Member							
	grandparents	father	mother	brother	sister	son	daughter	other
Colon or rectal cancer								
Other cancer								
Heart disease								
Diabetes								
High blood pressure								
Liver disease								
High cholesterol								
Alcohol/drug abuse								
Depression/psychiatric								
Genetic disorder								
Other								

SYMPTOM REVIEW

Gastrointestinal
- ☐ poor appetite
- ☐ abdominal pain
- ☐ indigestion
- ☐ trouble swallowing
- ☐ diarrhea
- ☐ constipation
- ☐ change in bowel habits
- ☐ nausea or vomiting
- ☐ rectal bleeding or blood in stools
- ☐ history of liver disease or abnormal liver tests

Cardiovascular
- ☐ chest pain
- ☐ history of angina or heart attack
- ☐ history of high blood pressure
- ☐ history of irregular beat
- ☐ history of poor circulation

Pulmonary/lungs
- ☐ shortness of breath
- ☐ persistent cough
- ☐ coughing up blood
- ☐ asthma or wheezing

Muscle/joint/bone
- ☐ swelling of ankles or legs pain, weakness or numbness in
- ☐ arms or hands
- ☐ back or hips
- ☐ legs or feet
- ☐ neck or shoulders

Neurologic
- ☐ history of stroke
- ☐ blackouts or loss of consciousness

General
- ☐ weight gain/loss of during last 6 months
- ☐ poor sleep
- ☐ fever
- ☐ headache
- ☐ depression

Eyes, ears, nose, throat
- ☐ blurred vision
- ☐ other change in vision
- ☐ history of glaucoma or cataracts
- ☐ loss of hearing
- ☐ ringing in ears
- ☐ sinus problems
- ☐ hoarseness

Genitourinary
- ☐ frequent or painful urination
- ☐ blood in urine

Skin
- ☐ itching
- ☐ easy bruising
- ☐ change in moles

Endocrine
- ☐ history of diabetes
- ☐ history of thyroid disease
- ☐ change in tolerance to hot or cold weather
- ☐ excessive thirst

Women only
- ☐ abnormal Pap smear
- ☐ bleeding between periods
  date of last mammogram _____

Men only
- ☐ PSA

Anything else?
- ☐ Are you experiencing an unusually stressful situation?
- ☐ Are there any specific personal issues you would like to bring up at the time of your visit?

Immunizations: if YES, give approximate year given

Pneumococcal No _____   Yes _____

Hepatitis A   No _____   Yes _____

Hepatitis B   No _____   Yes _____

Tetanus   No _____   Yes _____

Do you use seatbelts?   No _____   Yes _____

Transfusions: Have you ever received a blood transfusion? No _____ Yes _____ When? _____

The Clinical Medical Assistant Program

Handout #4

MEDICAL RECORDS

Purpose: Although a patient's healthcare record has numerous purposes, the most important of purpose is to help healthcare providers provide high quality and efficient patient care. The medical record is the repository of all the information about the patient related to patient care. Patient health record is now the standard term used for a collection of documents and other file types replacing patient medical record. The content varies depending upon whether the patient is in an outpatient facility or in an acute care facility. Health records can also be paper using traditional file storage systems and processes or more often electronic using electronic health record (EHR) software and systems.

Functions: There are many functions of the patient health record.

- The health record provides accurate information about the patient's treatment including health history information and information about any previous treatment.
- The health record provides the information used for billing the patient and insurance plans and for reimbursement to the providers.
- The health record serves as a legal document if there is ever a question of medical error. It becomes evidence in a court of law.
- The health record provides a basis for improvements in health and health maintenance.
- The health record provides data to many organizations including public health departments, law enforcement officials, and Homeland Security. The data is used to track births, deaths, communicable diseases, exposure to hazardous materials, bioterrorism threats, child abuse, and other crimes.
- The health record provides data to researchers for clinical trials, treatment and drug research, health trends, transplant and implant registries, and cancer registries.

Contents: The content and organization of the health record varies depending upon the medical specialty and whether the facility is an ambulatory facility or a hospital or other care facility. Explore the differences.

Acute Care Hospital	Doctor's Office
Registration Record	Registration Form
Consent Forms, Authorizations, Property List, Advance Directives	Consent Forms, Authorizations, Advance Directives
<ul><li>HIPAA Consent to Use and Disclose PHI</li><li>Consent to Treatment</li><li>Medicare Patient Rights Statement</li><li>Assignment of Benefits</li><li>Informed Consent</li><li>Refusal of Treatment</li><li>Advance Directives</li><li>Organ Donor</li><li>Personal Property List</li><li>Disclosure Records</li></ul>	<ul><li>HIPAA Consent to Use and Disclose PHI</li><li>Consent to Treatment</li><li>Medicare Patient Rights Statement</li><li>Assignment of Benefits</li><li>Informed Consent</li><li>Refusal of Treatment</li><li>Advance Directives</li><li>Disclosure Records</li></ul>
Medical History by the Admitting Doctor Physical Examination by the Admitting Doctor	Medical History from Patient Doctor's Notes (Encounter Notes) from each visit, organized by:
	<ul><li>Complaint</li><li>Symptoms</li><li>History</li><li>Review of Systems</li><li>Vital Signs</li><li>Physical Exam</li><li>Assessment</li><li>Plan of Care</li></ul>
Physician Orders Clinical Observations: Doctors' Notes, Nurses' Notes, Therapy Notes Surgery or Operative Report/Anesthesia Records Consultation Reports Test Results Discharge Summary Patient Discharge Instructions Case Management Reports	Diagnostic Test Orders and Test Results/Reports Flow Sheets (specialty specific, such as pediatrics, obstetrics, dermatology, etc.) Medical Records from Other Providers Consultation Reports Problem List Medication List Immunization Records Correspondence Authorization Forms to Disclose PHI Copies of Insurance Cards

Ownership of Health Records: The data of the patient record belongs to the patient; however, the actual patient record belongs to the facility or physician that created and maintains the records. HIPAA legislation assures that patients have the right to access, review, and request corrections to their health records.

Access to Health Records: Patients have the right to access and receive copies of their health records. Additionally, covered entities as described by HIPAA are authorized to access a patient's health records in order to provide patient care and conduct business related to that care, such as billing and reimbursement. Under HIPAA, a covered entity is a healthcare provider, a healthcare clearinghouse, and a health plan. Additionally, other entities, such as courts and public health departments, are authorized to access some of the data. Patients or courts may assign a personal representative to a patient who then becomes authorized to access the information. Parents and guardians of minor children also have authority to access the minor's health record in many, but not all, circumstances.

Storage and Destruction: Providers are required to maintain health records for a specific period of time. This requirement varies by medical profession and from state to state. Providers must also assure that the records are kept secure under HIPAA legislation. Providers may then destroy the records in a secure way after that time period.

The Clinical Medical Assistant Program

Handout #5

BODY MECHANICS

The Health Care Industry is facing a big challenge. Nursing personnel, orderlies and attendants have a risk of lost workday injuries and illnesses about 3.5 times that of the average private industry worker. Why are their rates high? Two words—back injuries. Health care workers are hurting their backs while lifting, transferring and otherwise moving patients or residents.

HOW WE ARE PUT TOGETHER

Back, neck, and shoulder injuries are the most frequent and costly type of injuries among health care workers. Some basic information on the structure and function of the body can help provide an understanding on how these injuries occur and how we can prevent them.

The Neck

The first seven vertebrae are called cervical vertebrae and form the neck. Areas of the spine such as the neck, where flexible and inflexible sections join, are particularly susceptible to strains, sprains and injuries.

The Shoulder

The shoulder is an example of a ball and socket joint where the ball of one bone fits into a hollow crevice of another. The shoulder joint allows movement and rotation of the arms inward, outward, forward or backward. There are several different tendons attached to bones in the shoulder. Bursae reduce friction and cushion the tendons as they slide back and forth.

The Back

The spine is a column of approximately 30 bones called vertebrae which run from the neck to the tailbone. These vertebrae are stacked on top of one another in an S-shaped column and form spinal joints which move independently. In the healthy spine there are three natural curves: a forward curve in the neck, a backward curve in the chest area, and another forward curve in the lower back. The back's three natural curves are correctly aligned when ears, shoulders and hips are in a straight line. At the end of the spine, the vertebrae are fused together to form the sacrum and the tailbone. The lower back or lumbar area is the workhorse of the back. It carries most of the weight and load of the body. Aligning and supporting the lumbar curve properly helps prevent injury to vertebrae, discs and other parts of the spine. The spine also has various types of associated soft tissues like the spinal cord, nerves, discs, ligaments, muscles and blood vessels.

Discs

Discs are soft, shock-absorbing cushions located between vertebrae. They allow vertebral joints to move smoothly and absorb shock as you move. Each disc has a spongy center (i.e., the nucleus pulposus) and tough outer rings (i.e., the annulus fibrosis).

Muscles and Ligaments Affecting the Back

The vertebrae are connected by a complex system of ligaments which "knit" them together. Strong flexible muscles maintain the three natural spinal curves and help in movement. The most important muscles which affect the spine are the stomach, hip flexors, hamstrings, buttock and back muscles.

Spinal Cord and Nerves

The spinal cord is a delicate cylinder of nerve fibers running the length of the spine inside a hollow tunnel formed by the vertebrae. Spinal nerves branch off of the spinal cord and exit through openings between vertebrae. These nerves then travel to all parts of the body.

Tendons

Tendons are tough, connective tissue that attaches muscles to bones. They help move the hands, arms, legs and other body parts by acting as "pulleys."

Bursae

Bursae are small sacs filled with fluid. They serve as soft slippery cushions between bony projections and muscle- tendon units.

TYPES OF INJURIES

Muscle Pain, Sprains and Strains

Pain in the muscles is extremely common. When muscles contract repetitively without sufficient rest they can become sore and painful. This can happen without movement (e.g., when holding objects or fixed body postures) or when we move repetitively. A sprain is damage to ligament fibers caused by moving or twisting a joint beyond its normal range. A strain occurs when a muscle or a muscle tendon unit is overused.

Bursitis

Bursitis is an irritation and inflammation of bursae in the shoulders and other areas caused by their rubbing on adjacent tendons.

Tendinitis and Tenosynovitis

When a tendon is overused, it can become inflamed and irritated causing tendonitis. When the tendon sheath is also involved, the condition is called tenosynovitis.

Neck Tension Syndrome

The joint where the last neck vertebra meets the first mid-back vertebra is a major site of acute back pain, muscle tension and other injuries. Common symptoms include: muscle tightness, soreness, restricted movement, headaches, numbness and tingling in the hands, wrists, arms or the upper back.

Shoulder Tendinitis, Bursitis and Impingement

Shoulder tendonitis is common in people who lift continuously or who work at levels above their shoulder. Several different tendons attach to bones in the shoulder region and produce different types of tendonitis, including rotator cuff and bicipital tendonitis. Shoulder bursitis inhibits the free movement of the tendons in the crowded shoulder girdle and limits the mobility of the shoulder. Shoulder impingement occurs when enlarged or inflamed bursae or tendons get caught between structures in the shoulder.

Degenerated, Bulging or Ruptured (Herniated) Discs

Over time, discs wear out or degenerate from natural aging. The discs dry out and become stiffer and less elastic. The outer fibrous rings can crack and the disc narrows. They become less able to handle loads put on them. If the inner jelly-like center bulges into the outer rings (i.e., the annulus), it may compress nearby nerves or blood vessels. If the inner jelly-like center breaks through the outer rings, the condition is called a ruptured (herniated) disc. The discs in the lower back are more susceptible to damage than other discs because they bear most of the load in lifting, bending and twisting.

Sciatica

Sciatica occurs when bulging or ruptured discs constrict the sciatic nerve or nearby blood vessels causing pain to be felt (i.e., referred) down the hips, buttocks or legs.

Wear and Tear Arthritis (Degenerative or Osteoarthritis)

Degenerative or "osteo" (bone) arthritis simply means the wearing out of joints, vertebrae, discs, facets or other structures over time. Osteoarthritis is associated with loads put on the spine over long time periods. As the discs dry out and narrow, they lose their shock-absorbing ability. The vertebrae become closer together, irritated and may produce bony outgrowths.

GUIDELINES FOR MANUAL LIFTING AND LATERAL TRANSFERS

Lifting

- Use upright, neutral working postures and proper body mechanics
- Bend your legs, not your back. Use your legs to do the work

- When lifting or moving people always face them
- Do not twist when turning. Pickup your feet and pivot your whole body in the direction of the move
- Try to keep the person you are moving, equipment and supplies close to the body. Keep hand-holds between your waist and shoulders
- Move the person towards you, not away from you
- Use slides and lateral transfers instead of manual lifting
- Use a wide, balanced stance with one foot slightly ahead of the other
- Lower the person slowly by bending your legs, not your back. Return to an erect position as soon as possible
- Use smooth movements and do not jerk. When lifting with others, coordinate lifts by counting down and synchronizing the lift

PROPER WORK PRACTICES

Lateral Transfers

- Position surfaces (e.g., bed and gurney, bed and cardiac chair) as close as possible to each other. Surfaces should be at approximately waist height, with the receiving surface slightly lower to take advantage of gravity
- Lower the rails on both surfaces (e.g., beds and gurneys)
- Use draw sheets or incontinence pads in combination with friction reducing devices (e.g., slide boards, slippery sheets, plastic bags, low friction mattress covers, etc.)
- Get a good hand-hold by rolling up draw sheets and incontenence pads or use other assist equipment such as slippery sheets with handles
- Kneel on the bed or gurney to avoid extended reaches and bending of the back
- Have team members on both sides of the bed or other surfaces. Count down and synchronize the lift.
- Use a smooth, coordinated push-pull motion. Do not reach across the person you are moving

GUIDELINES FOR AMBULATING, REPOSITIONING AND MANIPULATING

Using Gait or Transfer Belts with Handles

- Keep the individual as close as possible
- Avoid bending, reaching or twisting your back when:
- attaching or removing belts (e.g., raise or lower beds, bend at the knees)
- lowering the individual down
- assisting with ambulation
- Pivot with your feet to turn
- Use a gentle rocking motion to take advantage of momentum

Performing Stand-Pivot Type Transfers

- Used for transferring from bed to chair, etc., or to help an individual get up from a sitting position.
- Use transfer discs or other assists when available. If using a gait or transfer belt with handles, follow the above guidelines.
- Keep feet at least a shoulder width apart
- If the patient or resident is on a bed, lower the bed so that they can place their feet on the floor to stand

- Place the receiving surface (e.g., wheelchairs) on the individual's strong side (e.g., for stroke or hemiparalysis conditions) so they can help in the transfer
- Get the person closer to the edge of bed or chair and ask them to lean forward as they stand (if medically appropriate)
- Block the individual's weak leg with your legs or knees (this may place your leg in an awkward, unstable position; an alternative is to use a transfer belt with handles and straddle your legs around the weak leg of the patient or resident)
- Bend your legs, not your back
- Pivot with your feet to turn
- Use a gentle, rocking motion to take advantage of momentum

Lifting or Moving Tasks with the Patient or Resident in Bed

Some common methods include scooting up or repositioning individuals using draw sheets and incontinence pads in combination with a log roll or other techniques.

- Adjust beds, gurneys or other surfaces to waist height and as close to you as possible
- Lower the rails on the bed, gurney, etc., and work on the side where the individual is closest
- Place equipment or items close to you and at waist height
- Get help and use teamwork

GUIDELINES FOR TRANSPORTING PATIENTS, RESIDENTS AND EQUIPMENT

It is often necessary to transport people in gurneys, wheelchairs, or beds or handle various types of carts, monitors, instrument sets and other medical equipment.

- Decrease the load or weight of carts, instrument trays, etc.
- Store items and equipment between waist and shoulder height
- Use sliding motions or lateral transfers instead of lifting
- Push, don't pull. Keep loads close to your body. Use an upright, neutral posture and push with your whole body, not just your arms
- Move down the center of corridors to prevent collisions
- Watch out for door handles and high thresholds which can cause abrupt stops

GUIDELINES FOR PERFORMING ACTIVITIES OF DAILY LIVING

Cramped showers, bathrooms or other facilities in combination with poor work practices may cause providers to assume awkward positions or postures or use forceful exertions when performing ADLs.

- Use upright, neutral working postures and proper body mechanics. Bend your legs, not your back
- Eliminate bending, twisting and long reaches by using long-handled extension tools (e.g., hand-held shower heads, wash and scrub brushes)
- Wheeling people out of showers or bathrooms and turning them around to wash hard-to-reach places
- Use shower-toilet chairs which are high enough to fit over toilets. This eliminates additional transfers to and from wheelchairs, toilets, etc.

The Clinical Medical Assistant Program

Handout #6

PERIPHERAL INTRAVENOUS

A. The Three Types of Intravenous Fluids Are:

- Hypertonic solutions—Any solution that has a higher osmotic pressure than another solution (that is, has a higher concentration of solutes than another solution), which means it draws fluid out of the cell and into the extra-cellular space.
- Hypotonic solutions—Any solution that has a lower osmotic pressure than another solution (that is, has a lower concentration of solutes than another solution), which means it pushes fluid into the cell.
- Isotonic solutions—Any solution that has the same osmotic pressure than another solution (that is, has the same concentration of solutes than another solution), which means it does not draw or push fluid into the cell.

B. Commonly Used Intravenous Solutions:

- *Normal saline solution (NS, 0.9% NaCl)*—Isotonic solution (contains same amounts of sodium and chloride found in plasma). It contains 90 grams of sodium chloride per 100 ml of water. It is indicated for use in conjunction with blood transfusions and for restoring the loss of body fluids.
- *Ringer's Solution or Lactated Ringer's (LR)*—Isotonic solution (replaces electrolytes in amounts similarly found in plasma). It contains sodium chloride, potassium chloride, calcium chloride, and sodium lactate. It is indicated for use as the choice for burn patients, and in most cases of dehydration. It is also recommended for supportive treatment of trauma.
- *Five percent dextrose and water (D5W)*—Isotonic solution (after administration and metabolism of the glucose; D5W becomes a *hypotonic* solution). It contains 5 grams of dextrose per 100 ml of water. It is indicated for use as a calorie replacement solution and in cases where glucose is needed for metabolism purposes.
- *Five percent dextrose and ½ Normal Saline Solution (D51/2NS)*—Hypotonic solution that draws water out of the cells into the more concentrated extracellular fluid. Careful usage for

patients with cardiac or renal disease if they are unable to tolerate the extra fluid watch for pulmonary edema.

- *½ Normal Saline Solution*—Hypotonic solution that pushes fluid from the extracellular space into the cell. Watch if given to patients with increased ICP i.e. stroke, head trauma or neurosurgery.
- *TPN (total parenteral nutrition)*—TPN contains water, protein, carbohydrates (CHO), fats, vitamins, and trace elements that are necessary to the healing process. It is a very strong hypertonic solution. It must be given through a central venous catheter to allow rapid mixing and dilution.

C. Electrolytes

Multiple electrolyte solutions are helpful in replacing previous and concurrent fluid losses. Fluid and electrolyte losses that occur from diarrhea, vomiting, and/or gastric suction are an example of concurrent losses.

Nursing assessment for fluid volume deficit and fluid volume overload during IV therapy include:

FVD (Fluid Volume Deficit)
- Dry Skin (Capillary refill > 3 seconds)
- Elevated or Subnormal Temperature
- Thirst and Dry Mucus Membranes
- Decreased Urine Output
- Soft Sunken Eyeballs (> then 10% loss of total body fluid volume decreases intraocular pressure and cause eyes to appear to be sunken in)
- Decrease Tearing and Salivating
- Hypotension

FVO (Fluid Volume Overload)
- Pitting edema (1+ – 4+)
- Puffy eyelids
- Acute weight gain
- Elevated blood pressure
- Bounding pulse
- Dyspnea and shortness of breath (Usually first sign)
- Ascites or third spacing

Other nursing assessment observations that are important during IV therapy include:
- Close monitoring of weight gain/loss
- Accurate I and O (normal urine output is approximately 1 Ml/Kg of body wt. per hour)
- Assessing for signs of edema (skin that is tight and shiny)
- Assessing for skin turgor that when pinched takes longer then 3 seconds to return to normal.
- Assessing lung sounds (crackles will be heard with FVO)
- Notification to physician if urine output is < 30cc for two consecutive hours
- Monitor sodium and hematocrit levels

TYPES OF IV SOLUTIONS

Isotonic Saline (0.9%)

- Replaces sodium losses in conditions such as gastrointestinal fluid loss and burns.
- Contraindications are congestive heart failure, pulmonary edema, and renal impairment

Hypotonic Sodium Chloride 0.45%

- Hydrate cells and deplete the amount of fluid in the circulatory system
- No typical contraindications, added insulin for persons with diabetes mellitus

Isotonic 5% dextrose in water (D-5-W)

- Maintain fluid intake and provide daily caloric needs, acts as a peripheral nutrition, does not replace electrolyte deficiencies
- Contraindications are head injuries, added insulin for persons with diabetes mellitus

Isotonic Lactated Ringer's Solution and 5% Dextrose

- Has similar electrolytes as in plasma, correct metabolic acidosis, replaces fluid losses from conditions such as diarrhea and burns
- Contraindications are congested heart failure, renal impairment, liver disease, respiratory alkalosis acidosis

Hypotonic 5% dextrose in 0.9% NaCl

- Maintains fluid intake, is maintenance fluid of choice if no electrolytes are needed
- There are no typical contraindications, added insulin for persons with diabetes mellitus

Isotonic Lactated Ringers Solution

- Has similar electrolytes as in plasma, correct metabolic acidosis, replaces fluid losses from conditions such as diarrhea and burns
- Contraindications are congested heart failure, renal impairment, liver disease, respiratory alkalosis acidosis

STEPS TO STARTING A PERIPHERAL INTRAVENOUS

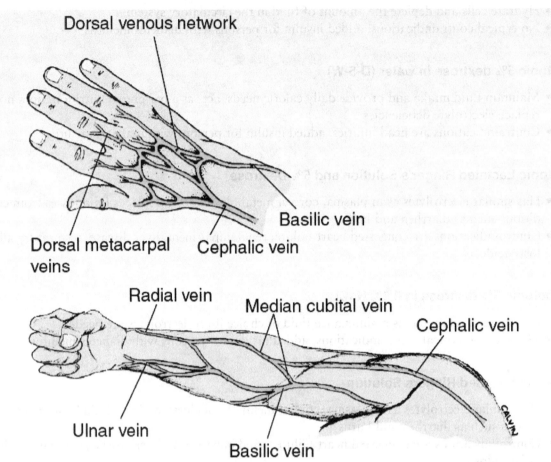

Superficial Veins of the Forearm and the Dorsal Aspect of the Hand

The flow of intravenous fluids is regulated by a roller clamp that is attached to the IV tubing. When the roller clamp is open fluids can infuse into the body at a rapid rate. As you close the roller clamp, the fluid will infuse at a slower rate.

A. Before Infusion

You will need the following supplies:

- _____ bag(s) of _____ (fluid to be infused)
- 1 microdrip tubing
- 1 30″ extension tubing

B. Setting Up Your Tubing

1. Wash your hands

2. Remove the microdrip tubing from the package. Straighten out the tubing.

3. Close the roller clamp.

4. Remove the 30″ extension tubing from its package. Attach the 30″ extension tubing to the end of the microdrib tubing.

5. Remove the rubber stopper from the IV bag.

6. Remove the cover from the spike of the microdrip tubing.
   DO NOT TOUCH THE END OF THE SPIKE.

7. Insert the spike into the IV bag.

8. Hang the IV bag from a pole.

9. Squeeze the drip chamber and release until fluid half fills the drip chamber.

10. Open the roller clamp. Allow the fluid from the bag to fill the entire IV tubing. Be certain that there are no air bubbles in the tubing.

11. Attach the IV tubing to your intravenous catheter.

C. IV Initiation (Cannulation)
Vein Selection

Most people learning to start IVs have struggles simply because they do not take the time to choose a good vein. Vein selection might be the single most important factor in 'getting' or 'missing' IVs. Additionally, choosing the appropriate vein can have an impact on patient care and outcome (see below). Here are some considerations when choosing veins.

- As a general principle, choose a vein that is most distal. Here's why: if you have an unsuccessful IV start (in non-technical terminology: if you blow a vein), then you cannot use a vein distal to the blown site because fluid or drug given at the distal site may still extravasate at the blown site. Also, reserving antecubital veins is helpful to hospital staff, which are required to take blood samples from these sites.
- Think of why the IV is being started. If a patient is in cardiac arrest, we do not care about choosing the most distal vein. We want to choose one that is as close to the patient's heart as possible and ideally is a large vein through which we could infuse fluids quickly. The antecubital veins become prime choices in the arrest situation. Similarly, Adenosine (treatment for SVTs) must be given from a site as close to the heart as possible.

- Choose a nice, 'juicy' vein. Veins that are easy to cannulate are prominent, feel spongy when palpated, and are big enough to accommodate the catheter.
- Avoid starting IVs anywhere on the hand or arm of a patient who:
    i. Has a fistula on that arm

    ii. Has lymphedema (a condition causing an accumulation of lymphatic fluid in interstitial spaces, most commonly in arms and legs) on that side. Any invasive procedure on the affected side may cause serious long-term damage to the arm.

    iii. Has had a radical mastectomy or blood clot on that side

    iv. Has a fracture or dislocation proximal to the site. You do not want to infuse fluids or drugs into the area via any damaged veins.

- Avoid insertion sites where there is bruising, scar tissue, disease, burns, etc. These will only cause you to "blow veins" more often.
- When possible, choose the right side first (truly a prehospital concern only). This is simply good practice because if you need to make additional attempts en route to hospital, the right arm is very difficult to access once your patient is in the vehicle. Starting an IV in the right antecubital fossa while in a moving ambulance requires awkward, mechanically unsound, potentially dangerous body positioning which is best avoided when possible.
- ⬜⬜ On obese patients, forearm veins will be nearly impossible to see or palpate, so look for hand veins first, then antecubital veins next.
- Avoid the anterior or palm side of the wrist. The radial nerve is very superficial, and insertion can be very painful for patients.
- ⬜⬜ Feet and leg veins are not good choices because of increased risk of thrombophlebitis and embolism.
- Choose a section of a vein that is straight. Your catheter is straight so it is a lot easier to advance it through a nice, straight vein.
- Starting IVs on pediatric patients is especially difficult because:
    i. Their veins are much smaller and less prominent.

    ii. They tend not to listen to your instructions to 'hold still' because they are petrified of any procedure that involves a needle.

D. Site Advantages/Disadvantages

Metacarpal Veins: Located on dorsum of hand; formed by union of digital veins
- Easily accessible
- Adapter lies flat on back of hand
- In adult or large child, bones of hand act as a splint
- Usually first choice for cannulation
- Wrist mobility decreased unless a short cannula is used
- Insertion painful because of large number of nerve endings
- Site becomes phlebitic more easily
- May be contraindicated with an aged patient as thin skin & loss of connective tissue may predispose to extravasation of blood

Basilic Vein: Runs along ulnar aspect of forearm & upper arm.
- Straight strong vein suitable for large-gauge cannula
- Uncomfortable position for patient during insertion
- Painful area to penetrate skin
- Vein tends to roll on insertion

Cephalic Vein: Runs along radial aspect of forearm and upper arm
- Large vein readily accepts large gauge cannula
- Does not impair mobility
- ⚠ ⚠ Decreases elbow joint mobility
- Vein tends to roll during insertion

Accessory Cephalic Vein: Runs along radius as a continuation of metacarpal veins of the thumb
- Large vein readily accepts large gauge cannula
- Does not impair mobility
- Does not require an arm board in older child or adult
- Sometimes difficult to position adapter flush with skin
- Adapter placed at bend of wrist, movement can cause discomfort or kinking of tubing

Antecubital Veins: Located in antecubital fossa (median cephalic, located on radial side; median basilic, on ulnar side; median cubital, in front of elbow joint)
- Often palpable or visible in children when other veins will not dilate
- May be used for peripheral IV therapy in an emergency or as a last resort
- Difficult to immobilize joint
- Median cephalic vein crosses in front of brachial artery, increasing the risk of arterial puncture and intra arterial infusion of medication resulting in permanent damage
- ⚠ ⚠ Veins may be small and scarred if blood has been drawn frequently

Median Antebrachial Vein: Arises from palm and runs along ulnar aspect of forearm
- A last resort when no other sites available
- ⚠ ⚠ Many nerve endings in area may cause painful venipuncture
- ⚠ ⚠ Infiltration occurs easily increasing risk of nerve damage

Digital Veins: Run along dorsal and lateral portions of fingers (digits)
- Last resort for fluid administration or for non-irritating medications
- Finger is splinted with a tongue depressor, limiting mobility
- Uncomfortable for patient
- ⚠ ⚠ Infiltration occurs very easily
- Cannot be used if metacarpal veins have already been used

E. Choosing the Gauge of the Catheter

Size does matter when it comes to choosing your IV catheter. It comes down to common sense. You choose a size appropriate for the situation and for the size of the vein. Larger bore IVs (18, 16, and 14) are appropriate for rapid infusion of fluids and/or blood and blood products but you need a big vein to get them in (and they hurt more). Additionally, putting a cannula into a vein that is too small can cause damage to that vein and put the patient at risk for phlebitis (because blood cannot easily flow around the catheter). Smaller bore IVs (20, 22, and 24) are adequate as a simple route for medication, and they are less painful. Blood can be given through a 20 or even a 22 gauge catheter, but it will be slower than if given through large bore catheters.

- 14 Gauge
  - Large adolescents or adult
  - Trauma
  - Rapid infusion of fluids and/or blood & blood products
  - Very painful insertion
  - Requires very large vein

- 16 Gauge
  - Adolescents and adults
  - Trauma
  - Infusion of large volume of fluids
  - Infusion of blood & blood products
  - Painful insertion
  - Requires large vein

- 18 Gauge
  - Older children, adolescents & adults
  - Fluid resuscitation
  - Infusion of blood, blood components & viscous solutions
  - Obstetric patients
  - Mildly painful insertion
  - Requires decent sized vein

- 20 Gauge
  - Children, adolescents & adults
  - Suitable for most infusions, TKVO lines
  - Infusion of blood or blood components
  - Commonly used
  - Slower to infuse large amounts of fluid

- 22 Gauge
  - Infants, toddlers, children, adolescents & adults (especially the aged & emaciated)
  - Suitable for most infusions
  - Easier to insert in small, thin, fragile veins
  - Use with slower flow rates
  - Difficult to insert into tough skin

- 24 Gauge
  - Neonates, infants, toddlers
  - Flow rate would be very slow

F. Prepare the Patient

Many patients are anxious about IV therapy. Recognition of the patient's feelings and education of the patient regarding the procedure, need and benefits is required. (Anxiety can cause vasoconstriction). Remember that a competent patient has the right to refuse the treatment.

G. Select the Equipment

Select the appropriate bag size of solution, administration set, and drip chamber. You will also need an IV catheter, alcohol swabs, clear sterile bandage (e.g., Tegaderm), a 2"x2" bandage for any spills or misses, skin tape, and tourniquet. Your sharps box should be positioned close by with an open lid.

H. Prepare the Solution Set

Ensure that the solution bag is the right type and size. Check the bag for clarity (no particulates or discoloration), integrity (no leaks when you squeeze the bag), and expiry date. Attach the administration set to the solution bag and prime (that is, run the IV solution through) the tubing. Usually, for macro drip lines, these are prepared before the call.

I. Select the Insertion Site

Raise the bed to a comfortable height (if the patient is on the bed) and adjust lighting as possible. Place the patient in a comfortable position with the extremity toward you. See 'Vein Selection' for more details.

J. Select the Cannulation Device

Use the device with the smallest diameter that allows correct administration of therapy. The catheter must always be smaller than the selected vein

K. Dilate & Palpate the Vein

Apply the tourniquet above the insertion site tight enough to restrict venous flow, while maintaining arterial flow. Try not to leave the tourniquet on for more than two minutes.

NOTE: if vasodilatation is not adequate, enhance it by:
- ⁇ Lowering arm below heart level
- Gently tapping vein with finger
- "Milking" vein away from tourniquet

L. Apply Gloves

M. Prepare the Site

Cleanse area with an appropriate disinfectant (usually an alcohol swab) in a circular motion from centre to periphery. Cleanse the area to a size equal to or larger than the bandage. Avoid palpation of the site after cleansing. Let the alcohol dry before you make your start or it really stings for the patient.

N. Insert the Cannulation Device

Ensure that the package was sealed. Remove the needle/cannula cap, holding the needle and cannula by the flash chamber. Inspect the cannulation device for imperfections (e.g., burrs, cracks, etc.). The plug on the flashback chamber should be tight, and the cannula should be able to spin on the needle (to ensure that it's not stuck to the needle—a manufacturing defect that happens occasionally). Anchor the vein by holding the skin taut below the site (really important). Point the needle in the direction of the blood flow and hold it at 10–30 degree angle with the bevel up. Keeping your hand steady, pierce the skin and vein. Look for a slow flow of dark blood moving into the flashback chamber.

O. Advancing the Cannulation Device

Decrease the angle of the needle almost parallel with the skin. Advance the catheter (and needle) about a half a centimeter (until you're sure the cannula itself, not just the needle, is in the vein). Now you have two choices to advance the cannula. You can hold the needle firmly and then advance the cannula off the needle. Or, you can withdraw the needle partially from the cannula, then advance the cannula.

NOTE: If you feel resistance, do NOT force the cannula. You may damage a valve. Withdraw the needle and cannula together. Withdrawing the cannula first may cut the cannula on the sharp needle and cause a piece of free flowing cannula to form a cannula embolus. Attempt venipuncture at another site with a new cannula

P. Release the Tourniquet

When the cannula is placed correctly, release the tourniquet.

Q. Withdraw the Needle

You should press firmly on the skin over the cannula tip to prevent bleeding on withdrawal. So long as you apply pressure to the right place, you need not stain anyone's plush white carpet. With the other hand, withdraw the needle and dispose of it in the sharps container. Attach the tubing.

R. Connect the Fluid Filled Tubing to Hub
Maintaining the cannula position let the fluid flow freely for 2–5 seconds to assure proper placement of the cannula. Observe for swelling indicating infiltration or leakage. (See "How to Troubleshoot an IV" for more details). Set the flow rate.

S. Apply Sterile Clear Dressing (e.g., Tegaderm)
Apply over insertion site and the cannula hub.

T. Tape the IV Tubing to the Skin
Avoid placing tape on the clear dressing. Keep in mind that curving it too tightly can kink the tubing.

U. Document the Procedure
Document the date, time, location and size of cannulation device, condition of site, number of attempts (if more than one attempt was required), type and amount of solution, and rate of infusion, and sign.

V. During Infusion
- Using a watch with a second hand, count the number of drops for one minute. Adjust the roller clamp so that _____ drops a minute infuse.
- Place a strip of tape next to the numbers of the IV bag.
- With a pen, mark the time of where the fluid should be after each hour.
- Observe the fluid level frequently and adjust the flow with the roller clamp as needed to be sure the fluid level is at the right time.
- For example, if the fluid is going in too fast, close the roller clamp slightly so that it will flow in at a slower rate.

W. Ending Infusion
- When the fluid level in the IV is almost at the end, close the roller clamp.
- If no further fluid is to be given, follow the instructions for capping, flushing, or decreasing the catheter. (See Capping, Flushing, and Decreasing sections of this manual for more information).
- If you are to infuse another bag of IV fluid, remove the rubber stopper from the new IV bag.
- Remove the old bag from the tubing and insert the spike of the tubing into the new bag.
- Follow steps #1 and #2 under care during infusion.
- If you receive fluids continuously 24 hours a day, the tubing must be changed every 48 hours.
- Follow steps 1 through 10 under the Setting Up Your Tubing heading in this section.
- Clamp the intravenous catheter. Disconnect the old IV tubing.
- Connect new IV fluid and tubing to the intravenous catheter. Proceed with instructions under Care During Infusion heading in this section.
- Remember: Don't touch the tip of your catheter or the tip of your IV tubing!

X. How to Troubleshoot an IV Infusion
- If an infusion is running too slowly or not at all, the problem may be easily corrected. It's helpful to start at the patient and work your way back to the IV bag. Check to see if:
- The site is edematous or leaking. Remove the cannula—it's likely interstitial.
- The cannula tip may be resting against the wall of the vein. Move the cannula slightly.
- The vein may be in spasm. Irritating or cold infusions may cause venous spasms. Apply a warm, moist towel to the arm to relieve spasm and increase the flow of the solution.
- The tape is too tight. Re-tape if needed.
- The tourniquet is still on. Remove it.
- The joint above the site is flexed. Reposition the extremity or splint with an arm board.
- The tubing is dangling below the site. Gravity may be preventing flow. Reposition the tubing.

- The tubing is kinked, curved too tightly, or caught under the patient. Untangle the tubing. Use a firm "loop" to prevent tight curves at the cannula, and/or reposition the patient.
- The clamp is closed or has crimped the tubing. Move it to a different position on the tubing and recalculate the rate.
- The solution container is less that 90 cm (3 feet) above the site. Raise the IV pole.
- The bag is empty. Replace it.

If you are still unable to correct the rate of flow, restart the intravenous in the opposite hand or upper arm if possible.

PREPARING THE ADULT PATIENT FOR A PERIPHERAL IV

Many patients feel apprehensive about peripheral IV therapy. Before you begin therapy, teach the patient what to expect before, during, and after the procedure. Thorough patient teaching can reduce his anxiety, making therapy easier. Follow the guidelines below:

- Tell the patient that "intravenous" means "inside the vein" and that a plastic catheter (plastic tube) or needle will be placed in his vein. Explain that fluids containing certain nutrients or drugs will flow from an IV bag or bottle through a length of tubing, and then through the plastic catheter or needle in their vein.
- If you know about how long the catheter or needle will stay in place, tell the patient. Explain that the physician will decide how much and what type of fluid he needs.
- Mention that he may feel some pain during the insertion but that the discomfort will stop once he catheter or needle is in place.
- Tell him that the IV fluid may feel cold at first but this sensation should only last a few minutes.
- Explain that removing a peripheral IV line is a simple procedure. Let them know that once the IV is removed, pressure will be applied until the bleeding stops. Reassure him that, once the device is out and the bleeding stops he will be able to use their arm as usual.
- Tell the patient to report any discomfort after the catheter/needle has been inserted and the fluid has begun to flow.
- Explain any restrictions. If appropriate, tell the patient he can walk while receiving therapy. Depending on the insertion site, he may also be able to shower or take a tub bath during therapy.
- Teach the patient how to assist in IV system care. Tell him not to pull at the insertion site or tubing and not to remove the container from the IV pole. Also tell him not to kink the tubing or lie on it. Explain that he should call the nurse if the infusion rate suddenly slows down or speeds up.

PREPARING THE CHILD/INFANT PATIENT FOR A PERIPHERAL IV

- Child will need emotional support and reassurance.
- Explain to the child what to expect with the procedure (developmentally appropriate).
- Inserting the IV can be painful and frightening, the child may not understand why the IV is required.
- Select a neutral place for the IV start—perform the procedure in the treatment room. This ensures that the patient's room remains a "safe place" that is not associated with pain or frightening procedures.
- If the child cries during the procedure, let them know that it is OK to cry, but try to explain to them the need to remain still-encourage slow deep breaths, counting, looking the other way . . .

- Praise the child during and after the procedure.
- Keep the child warm-especially important for neonates and premature babies-use overhead radiant heater if applicable.

Positioning

- Discuss different options with the parent and child.
- Use restraints only if necessary.
- The height of the bed should facilitate the nurse's comfort.
- Do not attempt to do the procedure without assistance—it would be a mistake to assume that the child will not loose control even if they promise to cooperate.
- Neonate:
  - Swaddle securely or have a 2nd nurse assist in supporting the infant.
  - Minimize pain and discomfort by performing the procedure quickly and efficiently.
  - Consider infant positioning needs when choosing the IV site—avoid antecubital sites if infant requires prone positioning.
  - Facilitate hand-to-mouth activity.
- Infants:
  - Swaddle or mummy wrap, leaving the extremity of choice out.
  - If veins do not fully distend sufficiently, remove the tourniquet and allow the vessels to refill. Sometimes veins will fill better on the second try due to rebound effect.

1. Arm dangling—dangling the arm over the side of the bed may also assist in vein dilation

2. Gentle tapping—gentle tapping or flicking the veins with a finger will assist in vasodilation. Do not slap the skin.

3. Relaxation—a frightened or anxious patient may readily vasoconstrict. Help the patient to relax with techniques such as deep breathing or distractions

4. Heat—rub or stroke to warm skin, warm towels may be applied to promote vasodilation

SPECIAL CONSIDERATIONS FOR NEONATAL AND PEDIATRIC PATIENTS

Preparation of the parent/caregiver

- Explain to the parents what to expect with the procedure.
- Assess the child's past experience with an IV—it may be helpful to ask them or their parents what worked well the last time.
- Parents need to be informed why an IV is required, how long it may be needed and a basic review of how the IV works.
- The parents should be given the option of remaining with the child or leaving.
- If the parent chooses to stay with their child encourage them to provide support and comfort to their child—holding of hand, talking with the child, distracting activity.
- Parents should discuss coping strategies prior to the procedure—will hold parents hand, looking the other way.
- Do not assume the parent will be your assistant to help secure the child unless they choose to—instruct the parent on proper technique to secure the child.
- Reassure the parents that the child can still be active and play with the IV in place.

- Encourage parents to continue to provide care for their child—nurse needs to demonstrate how best to hold their infant who has an IV.
- Instruct parents in what to look for and when to call a nurse to assess the IV, this may include—IV pump alarming, leaking fluid or blood at the site, any redness or swelling noted at the insertion site.

RATE OF FLOW

I. FACTORS INFLUENCING RATE

Correcting obvious flow rate problems:

When your patient's infusing is running too slowly, or not at all, problems may be easily corrected. Begin by looking for the obvious. Then check to see if:
- The container's empty. If it is, replace it.
- The drip chamber's less than half full. Squeeze it until the fluid reached the proper level.
- The flow clamp's closed. Readjust to restore proper drip rate.
- The tubing is kinked or caught under the patient. Untangle the line and reposition patient
- The container is less than 3 feet above the site. Readjust the height of the IV pole.
- The tubing is dangling below the site and gravity is preventing the solution from reaching the patient. To remedy this problem, replace the tubing with a shorter piece, or tape some of the excess tubing to the IV pole (just below the flow clamp). If you tape the tubing, make sure you don't kink it accidentally.
- An air bubble is in the tubing. Tap the tubing until the bubble rises into the container.

II. CORRECTING FLOW RATE PROBLEMS

- If the IV isn't running at the prescribed rate, sometimes a clot is in the needle blocking the infusion. Close the flow clamp, and try aspirating the clot with a syringe on the catheter hub. Never try irrigating a clogged IV with a syringe and solution. You will increase the chance of infection and risk propelling the clot into the bloodstream.
- If the infusion is running sluggishly, the needle or catheter may be jammed against the vein wall. Be careful not to puncture the vein with the bevel triggering infiltration or thrombophlebitis.
- In some cases, you can restore the flow by changing the angle of the needle or catheter. To do this, elevate it slightly with a sterile 2 x 2 gauze.
- Occasionally you may discover that the infusion is running too quickly. Look first for a soaked dressing. This usually means that the needle or catheter has worked out of the skin underneath the dressing.
- Another way to revive a sluggish IV is by pinching the tubing near the IV site. If the line includes a flashbulb, compress it once or twice.

COMPLICATIONS IN IV THERAPY

A. Infiltration

An accumulation of fluid in the tissue surrounding an IV Catheter site. It is usually caused by penetration of the vein wall by the catheter itself and later leads to dislodgement out of the vein and into the tissue.

Signs and systems of infiltration include:
- Flow rate may either slow significantly or completely stop (IV Pump will "beep" occlusion)
- Infusion site becomes cool and hard to the touch
- Infusion site or extremity may become pale and swollen

- Patient may complain of pain, tenderness, burning or irritation at the IV site
- There may be noted fluid leakage around the site

Immediate corrective action to take if IV infiltration is suspected includes:
- Stop IV infusion immediately and remove IV Catheter
- Elevate extremity
- If noticed within 30 minutes of onset, apply ice to the site (this will decrease inflammation)
- If noticed later then 30 minutes of onset apply warm compress (this will encourage absorption)
- Notify Supervisor/Physician as per individual hospital policy
- Document findings and actions
- Restart IV in an alternative location (opposite extremity if possible)

Preventive measures to avoid IV infiltration include:
- Properly securing catheter hub to the limb
- Stabilize extremity in use by applying an arm board if necessary
- Frequent assessment of IV site
- Keep flow rate at the prescribed rate
- Change IV site and tubing per hospital policy

B. Phlebitis
Inflammation of the wall of the vein, usually caused by:
- Injury to vein during puncture
- Later movement of the catheter
- Irritation to the vein from long term therapy
- Vein overuse
- Irritating or incompatible solutions
- Large bore IVs
- Lower extremity IVs (greater risk)
- Infection

Signs and symptoms of phlebitis include:
- Sluggish flow rate
- Swelling around infusion site
- Patient complaint of pain or discomfort at site
- Redness and warmth along vein

Prevention and treatment for phlebitis is the same for an infiltrated IV.

C. Air Embolism
An air embolism is the obstruction of a blood vessel (usually occurring in the lungs or heart) by air carried via the bloodstream. The minimum quantity of air that may be fatal to humans is not known. Animal experimentation indicates that fatal volumes of air are much larger than the quantity present in the entire length of IV tubing. Average IV tubing holds about 5 ml of air, an amount not ordinarily considered dangerous.

Causes of air embolism include:
- Failure to remove air from IV tubing
- Allowing solution bags to run dry
- Disconnecting IV tubing

Signs and symptoms of air embolism include:
- Abrupt drop in blood pressure
- Weak, rapid pulse

- Cyanosis
- Chest pain

Immediate corrective action for suspected air embolism includes:
- Notify Supervisor and Physician immediately
- Immediately place patient on left side with feet elevated (this allows pulmonary artery to absorb small air bubbles)
- Administer O2 if necessary

Preventive measures to avoid air embolism includes:
- Clear all air from tubing before attaching it to the patient
- Monitor solution levels carefully and change bag before it becomes empty
- Frequently check to assure that all connections are secure

Complications	Signs and Symptoms	Purpose
Circulatory overload	• Neck vein distention or engorgement • Respiratory distress • Increased blood pressure • Positive fluid balance	• Stop infusion and place patient in semi-fowler's position, as tolerated • Reduce the patient's anxiety • Administer oxygen • Notify the physician • Administer diuretics • Monitor patient's vital signs
Hypersensitivity	• Itching, uticarial rash • Tearing eyes, runny nose • Bronchospasm • Wheezing • Anaphylactic reaction	• Stop the infusion • Maintain a patent airway • Administer an antihistaminic steroid, an anti-inflammatory drug or an antipyretic • Give 0.2 to 0.5 if 1:1000 aqueous epinephrine sub Q; repeat at 3 minute intervals as needed • Monitor the patient's vital signs
Infiltration	• Swelling • Discomfort • Burning • Tightness • Cool skin • Blanching	• Stop the infusion and remove the device (unless drug is a vesicant, in such cases consult the pharmacy) • Elevate the limb • Check the patient's pulse and capillary refill • Restart the IV • Document patient's condition • Check site frequently
Phlebitis	• Redness or tenderness at the tip of the device • Puffy area over the vein • Elevated temperature	• Stop the infusion and remove the device • Apply a warm pack • Document the patient's condition and interventions • Insert a new IV catheter using a larger vein or a smaller device

Complications	Signs and Symptoms	Purpose
Systemic infection	• Elevated temperature • Malaise	• Stop the infusion • Notify the physician • Remove the device • Culture the site and device • Administer meds as ordered • Monitor patient's vital signs
Venous spasm	• Pain along the vein • Sluggish flow rate when clamp is completely open • Blanched skin over vein	• Apply warm soaks over the vein and surrounding tissue • Slow the flow rate
Speed shock	• Headache • Syncope • Flushed face • Tightness in chest • Irregular pulse • Shock • Cardiac arrest	• Stop the infusion • Call the physician • Give dextrose 5% in water and keep the vein open rate

PREVENTING IV DRUG INCOMPATIBILITIES

The compatibility or incompatibility of IV medication is an important consideration in drug administration, especially since it is not unusual for multiple drugs to be administered through y-site connectors on continuous infusion administration sets. Even if patients are receiving different medications through multiple lumens of central venous catheters, care must be taken to assure that drugs administered into the same lumen are compatible.

Let's look at the different kinds of medication incompatibilities:

- **Visual:** A visual incompatibility is characterized by the presence of precipitation (visible particles seen floating in the solution), gas formation (solutions may appear carbonated), color change (drug references will tell you the correct appearance of an admixed medication in a solution), or turbidity, where medications do not mix easily into solution.
- **Chemical:** This often involves the degradation of drugs to produce therapeutically inactive or even toxic solutions. Chemical incompatibilities may not be accompanied by any visible clues.
- **Equivocal Compatibility:** Compatibility is reported as equivocal in situations in which signs of possible incompatibility are transient (such as turbidity that is resolved during a short time period, uncertain, or inconsistent).
- **Solution Instability:** This is when a medication comes out of solution or degrades due to the length of time it has been admixed or some other factor, such as temperature, or light exposure. Other factors influencing solution stability are the dose and concentration of the drug, the number, type, and order of additives to a solution, the type and volume of parenteral solution (for example, the electrolyte content of many parenteral nutrition solutions can alter the stability of most IV medications. This is an example of complexation, where two or more compounds in a solution form a chemical complex that inactivates one or both of them).
- **Therapeutic Incompatibility:** The largest class of incompatibilities is therapeutic incompatibility, which occurs when an undesirable pharmacological reaction occurs within the patient as a result of two or more incompatible medications concurrently. These medications do not necessarily

have to be given via the same route. It is imperative that the pharmacy be aware of ALL medications, dietary supplements, and over the counter medications that a patient has been taking in order to prevent known therapeutic incompatibilities.

To prevent incompatibilities, it is important to consider all the ways in which medications may interact outside of or inside the body. If you must mix a medication, always follow manufacturer's instructions as to the correct volume and type of diluent; which solutions it may be added to for "piggy back" administration; and what flush solutions must be used in between administrations to prevent events like precipitation within the patient's access device (for example, never administering phenytoin into an intravenous line containing dextrose, or never allowing amphotericin B to come into contact with saline solutions). Other issues to consider are the presence of electrolytes (e.g. potassium chloride) mixing into continuous infusions, such as in a piggyback situation. If mixing medications in a syringe for bolus administration (IV push), assure that they are compatible when combined in a syringe. If consulting a drug reference is not helpful, contact the pharmacy, which has access to additional compatibility information.

Be on alert for medications with a known history of frequent incompatibilities when they come into contact with other drugs. Among the drugs most often incriminated in incompatibilities are furosemide (Lasix), phenytoin (Dilantin), heparin, midazolam (Versed), and diazepam (Valium) when used in IV admixtures.

The Clinical Medical Assistant Program

Handout #7

NHA CCMA CERTIFICATION REVIEW GUIDE

See Attachment:
NHA CCMA Certification Review Guide

PART C
Clinical Medical Assistant

CLASSROOM SKILLS SUMMARY

CLINICAL MEDICAL ASSISTANT SKILLS SUMMARY
TO BE PERFORMED IN CLASSROOM—LABS AND DISCUSSIONS - 9/27/11

Skill #	SKILL DESCRIPTION	Page #	Lab Performed in Class	Discussion in Class
	CLINICAL MEDICAL ASSISTING SKILLS ("CMA Text")			
6-1	Prepare and Maintain the Medical Record	66		X
6-2	Complete a History Form	70	X	
6-3	Document a Clinical Visit and Procedure	74		X
7-1	Handwashing	88		X
7-2	Non-Sterile Gloving	90	X	
8-1	Sanitization	98		X
8-2	Disinfection	101		X
8-3	Wrapping Surgical Instruments for Autoclave Sterilization	104		X
8-4	Loading and Operating an Autoclave	105		X
8-5	Opening a Sterile Surgical Pack to Create a Sterile Field	107		X
8-6	Transfer Forceps	108		X
8-7	Performing a Surgical Scrub	109		X
8-8	Sterile Gloving and Glove Removal	112		X
9-1	Demonstrate the Preparation of a Prescription for the Physician's Signature	129		X
9-2	Demonstrate Withdrawing Medication from an Ampule	133		X
9-3	Withdrawing Medication from a Vial	134	X	
9-4	Demonstrate the Reconstitution of a Powdered Drug for Injection Administration	136		X
9-5	Demonstrate the Administration of Medication During Infusion Therapy	137		X
9-6	Preparation and Administration of Oral Medication	138	X	
9-7	Administration of Subcutaneous Injection	140	X	
9-8	Administration of Intramuscular Injection	141	X	
9-9	Demonstrate the Administration of a Z-Tract Injection	142		X
10-1	Obtain an Oral Temperature with an Electronic Digital Thermometer	151	X	

Skill #	SKILL DESCRIPTION	Page #	Lab Performed in Class	Discussion in Class
10-2	Obtain an Axillary Temperature with an Electronic Digital Thermometer	152		X
10-3	Obtain a Rectal Temperature with an Electronic Digital Thermometer	153		X
10-4	Obtain Aural Temperature	154	X	
10-5	Obtain a Dermal Temperature with a Disposable Thermometer	156		X
10-6	Perform Radial Pulse	158	X	
10-7	Perform a Apical Pulse Count	159	X	
10-8	Perform Respiration Count	160	X	
10-9	Measure Blood Pressure	163	X	
10-10	Obtain Weight and Height Measurements	165		X
10-11	Demonstrate Patient Positions Used in Medical Examinations	169		X
10-12	Assist the Physician with the Physical Exam	172		X
11-1	Prepare the Skin for Surgical Procedure	183		X
11-2	Set Up a Sterile Tray and Assist the Physician with Minor Surgical Procedures	186		X
11-3	Assist the Physician with Suturing	191		X
11-4	Assist the Physician with Suture or Staple Removal	192		X
11-5	Change a Sterile Dressing	196		X
16-1	Perform General Procedure for X-ray Examination	309		X
16-2	Filing and Loaning Radiographic Records	320		X
18-1	Demonstrate Performance of Spirometry	374		X
18-2	Demonstrate Performance of Peak Flow Testing	376		X
18-3	Demonstrate Performance of the Mantoux Test	377		X
18-4	Demonstrate Patient Instruction in the Use of an Inhaler	380		X
18-5	Demonstrate Patient Assistance in the Use of a Nebulizer	381		X
19-1	Measure Distance Visual Acuity with a Snellen Chart	395	X	
19-2	Perform the Ishihara Color Vision Test	396		X
19-3	Perform Eye Irrigation	397		X

Skill #	SKILL DESCRIPTION	Page #	Lab Performed in Class	Discussion in Class
19-4	Perform Instillation of Eye Medication	398		X
19-5	Perform Simple Audiometry	403		X
19-6	Perform Ear Irrigation	404		X
19-7	Perform Instillation of Ear Medication	405		X
23-1	Perform Adult Rescue Breathing and One-Rescuer CPR	468		X
23-2	Use an Automated External Defibrillator (AED)	470		X
23-3	Respond to an Adult with an Obstructed Airway	472		X
23-4	Administer Oxygen	476		X
23-5	Demonstrate Application of a Pressure Bandage	478		X
23-6	Demonstrate the Application of Triangular Sling	482	X	
23-7	Demonstrate the Application of a Splint	489		X
24-1	Assist with a Colon Endoscopic/Colonoscopy Exam	521		X
24-2	Assist with a Sigmoidoscopy	522		X
24-3	Insert a Rectal Suppository	523		X
25-1	Fiberglass Cast Application	544		X
25-2	Cast Removal	546		X
25-3	Assist the Patient with Cold Application/Cold Compress	548		X
25-4	Assist the Patient with Hot Moist Application/Hot Compress	549		X
25-5	Therapeutic Ultrasonography	550		X
25-6	Demonstrate Measuring for Axillary Crutches	551		X
25-7	Crutch Walking	555		X
25-8	Using a Cane	556		X
25-9	Using a Walker	557		X
25-10	Assist a Patient in a Wheelchair to and from an Exam Table	559		X
26-1	Prenatal Exam	574		X
26-2	Breast Self-Exam	579		X
26-3	Pelvic Exam and PAP	580		X
26-4	Urine Pregnancy Test	583		X
26-5	Assist with Cryosurgery	584		X

Skill #	SKILL DESCRIPTION	Page #	Lab Performed in Class	Discussion in Class
27-1	Perform and Record Measurements of Height or Length, Weight, and Head and Chest Circumference	593		X
27-2	Perform and Record Pediatric Vital Signs and Vision Screening	595		X
27-3	Perform documentation of Immunization, Both Stored and Administered	597		X
27-4	Perform Urine Collection with a Pediatric Urine Collection Bag	605		X
28-1	Assist with a Neurological Exam	615		X
28-2	Assist with a Lumbar Puncture	616		X
28-3	Prepare a Patient for an Electroencephalogram	617		X
31-1	—Role-Play Sensormotor Changes of the Elderly	659		X

Note: The page references above are pages in the Textbook which provide instructions for completing the above tasks in the classroom.

PART D
Clinical Medical Assistant

STUDENT GRADUATE ASSISTANCE PACKET

TABLE OF CONTENTS

Topic   Page

Introduction D-3

The Resume D-4

The Interview D-11

Interview Follow Up D-15

The Job Search D-17

Note: This packet can be used by students interested in finding employment in health care as well as other related fields. The information in this packet includes helpful hints, best practices, interview techniques and other information to assist students in their search for life-long employment.

The Clinical Medical Assistant Program

INTRODUCTION

Your hands are damp as you wring them uncontrollably. Your mouth is dry, and you wonder if the right words will ever escape you lips. Your stomach is doing loop-de-loops as you make yet another run for the bathroom. And this is only the day before the interview!

Does this sound like you? You're not alone. It is very common, and normal, to be nervous before an interview. Feeling anxious will raise your energy level, and that's a good thing, just be sure you don't get too nervous. The best way to avoid common job search and interview mistakes is to prepare.

The Clinical Medical Assistant Program

THE RESUME

Your resume is a tool with one specific purpose: to win an interview. A resume is an advertisement, nothing more, nothing less.

A great resume doesn't just tell them what you have done but makes the same assertion that all good ads do: If you buy this product (Me), you will get these specific, direct benefits. It presents you in the best light. It convinces the employer that you have what it takes to be successful in this new position or career.

It is so pleasing to the eye that the reader is enticed to pick it up and read it. It "whets the appetite," stimulates interest in meeting you and learning more about you. It inspires the prospective employer to pick up the phone and ask you to come in for an interview.

Your cover letter should make the reader want to learn more about you and provide a preview to your resume. It should not provide the same details as your resume but act as an introduction to your resume.

When creating your resume, use the following guidelines:

- **The resume is visually enticing,** a work of art. Simple clean structure. Very easy to read . . . Uncrowded.
- **There is uniformity and consistency in the use of italics, capital letters, bullets, boldface, and underlining.** For example, if a period is at the end of one job's dates, a period should be at the end of all jobs' dates.
- **There are absolutely no errors.** No typographical errors. No spelling errors. No grammar, syntax, or punctuation errors. No errors of fact.
- **All the basic, expected information is included.** A resume must have the following key information: your name, address, phone number, and your email address at the top of the first page, a listing of jobs held, in reverse chronological order, educational degrees including the highest degree received, in reverse chronological order. Additional, targeted information will of course accompany this.

- **Jobs listed** include a title, the name of the firm, the city and state of the firm, and the years.
- **It is targeted.** A resume should be targeted to your goal, to the ideal next step in your career.
- **Strengths are highlighted/weaknesses de-emphasized.** Focus on whatever is strongest and most impressive.
- **Use power words.** For every skill, accomplishment, or job described, use the most active impressive verb you can think of (which is also accurate).
- **Show you are results-oriented.** Wherever possible, prove that you have the desired qualifications through a clear strong statement of accomplishments . . . For example: "Initiated and directed complete automation of the Personnel Department, resulting in time-cost savings of over 25%."
- **Writing is concise and to the point.** Keep sentences as short and direct as possible.
- **Make it look great.** Use a laser printer or an ink jet printer that produces high-quality results. Use a standard conservative typeface (font) in 11 or 12 point. Don't make them squint to read it. Use off-white, ivory or bright white 8 1/2 × 11-inch paper, in the highest quality affordable.
- **Shorter is usually better.** Everyone freely gives advice on resume length. Most of these self-declared experts say a resume should always be one page.
- **Break it up.** A good rule is to have no more than six lines of writing in any one writing "block" or paragraph (summary, skill section, accomplishment statement, job description, etc.). If any more than this is necessary, start a new section or a new paragraph.
- **Experience before education . . . usually.** Experience sections should come first, before education, in most every case.
- **Telephone number that will be answered.** Be sure the phone number on the resume will, without exception, be answered by a person or an answering machine Monday through Friday 8 AM–5 PM.

EMPLOYMENT HISTORY GAPS

"What's wrong with a few gaps in my work history?" you might ask. "Isn't everyone entitled to a little time off?" Many responsible professionals have taken breaks in their careers to travel, take care of ill parents, recover from illness, and a myriad of other legitimate projects. But for some reason, employers don't like to see gaps in your work history.

If you have a period of unemployment in your history, here are some ways of dealing with it:

1. Use only years, not months, when referring to spans of time in your work history. This makes it quicker for the reader to grasp the length of time, and can eliminate the need to explain some gaps that occurred within two calendar years.

2. If your unemployment covers two calendar years or more, you need to explain the void. Consider all the things you were doing (volunteer work, school activities, internships, schooling, and travel) during that time and present them in terms that are relevant to your job objective if possible.

3. If your gap has no apparent relevance to your job objective, explain the gap honestly and with dignity. References to illness, unemployment (even if it is clearly due to a recession), and rehabilitation raise red flags in most cases, so avoid those at all cost. Speak about something else that you were doing during that time, even if it doesn't relate to your job objective. Suggested "job titles":
   - Full-time Parent
   - Home Management
   - Family Management
   - Family Financial Management
   - Independent Study
   - Personal Travel

WHAT NOT TO PUT ON A RESUME

- The word "Resume" at the top of the resume
- Fluffy rambling "objective" statements
- Salary information
- Full addresses of former employers
- Reasons for leaving jobs
- A "Personal" section, or personal statistics (except in special cases)
- Names of supervisors
- References

ACCURACY/HONESTY/STRETCHING THE TRUTH

Make sure that you can back up what you say. Keep the claims you make within the range of your own integrity. There is nothing wrong with pumping things up in your resume so that you communicate who you are and what you can do at your very best.

SOME ADDITIONAL ADVICE

1. Your resume is about your future; not your past.

2. It is not a confessional. In other words, you don't have to "tell all." Stick to what's relevant and marketable.

3. Don't write a list of job descriptions. Write achievements!

4. Promote only skills you enjoy using. Never write about things you don't want to repeat.

5. Be honest. You can be creative, but don't lie.

Your name
Mailing address
City, state, and zip
Telephone number(s)
Email address

Today's date

Your addressee's name
Professional title
Organization name
Mailing address
City, state and zip

Dear Mr. (or Ms.) last name,

Start your letter with a grabber—a statement that establishes a connection with your reader, a probing question, or a quotable quote. Briefly say what job you are applying for.

The mid-section of your letter should be one or two short paragraphs that make relevant points about your qualifications. You should not summarize your resume! You may incorporate a column or bullet point format here.

Your last paragraph should initiate action by explaining what you will do next (e.g., call the employer) or instigate the reader to contact you to set up an interview. Close by saying "thank you."

Sincerely yours,

Your handwritten signature

Your name (typed)

Enclosure: resume

Your Name
Address
Telephone #

Date

Dear _____,

I am pleased to submit this resume as application for the _____ position available with your company.

Since graduating from the _____ course at (the college name), I have continued to expand my skills and am currently preparing for the _____ certification exam.

I strive to perform to the best of my ability and my work ethic is based on being a conscientious, honest, and reliable employee. I believe that the training I have received as well as my compassion for the patient will enable me to become a productive team member with your company.

I truly enjoy helping people. This is one of the greatest assets I can bring to your company. This passion is reflected in my performance and contributes greatly to my success as well as the quality of care received by my patients.

Thank you for your time and consideration.

Respectfully,

[Your Name]
[Street Address], [City, ST ZIP Code]
[phone]
[e-mail]

Objective	*Medical Assistant/Technologist position for a private practice.*

Professional Experience	**Patient Service Technician/Unit Clerk** OAK TREE COMMUNITY HOSPITAL, Coronary Care Unit, Columbus, Indiana • Order lab work and x-rays • Prioritize patient daily care according to acuity and scheduled patient procedures • Assist patients with A.M. care, take vital signs, prep for procedures, draw blood, and obtain specimens • Maintain and set up patient rooms • Perform preventive maintenance on emergency equipment • Assist with patient and family education • Assist R.N. with sterile and non-sterile dressing changes • Perform EKGs • Trained in Phlebotomy • Utilize PC to enter and retrieve patient data • Answer multi-line phone, operate fax and copy machine **Office Assistant,** (6-month part-time position) GARTH FORT, M.D., Columbus, Indiana • Answered phone, scheduled patients • Greeted patients • Updated patient charts

Education	In-house training programs, *Oak Tree Community Hospital* EKG, 1993 Phlebotomy, 1993 Tech Class, 1992 Unit Clerk Class, 1990 Nursing Assistant Class, 1989 CPR Certified, since 1989 *Elm Tree Community College* Computer training: WordPerfect I, Certificate 1995 *Maple Grove State University* Major: Pre-Veterinarian, 1989–1990

POWER WORDS

Accomplish	Delegate	Innovate	Publish
Achieve	Demonstrate	Inspect	Qualify
Act	Design	Install	Raise
Adapt	Detail	Institute	Recommend
Administer	Determine	Instruct	Reconcile
Advertise	Develop	Integrate	Record
Advise	Devise	Interpret	Recruit
Aid	Direct	Interview	Rectify
Analyze	Distribute	Introduce	Redesign
Apply	Draft	Invent	Reduce
Approach	Edit	Investigate	Regulate
Approve	Employ	Lead	Relate
Arrange	Encourage	Maintain	Renew
Assemble	Enlarge	Manage	Report
Assess	Enlist	Manipulate	Represent
Assign	Establish	Market	Reorganize
Assist	Estimate	Mediate	Research
Attain	Evaluate	Moderate	Resolve
Budget	Examine	Modify	Review
Build	Exchange	Monitor	Revise
Calculate	Execute	Motivate	Scan
Catalogue	Exhibit	Negotiate	Schedule
Chair	Expand	Obtain	Screen
Clarify	Expedite	Operate	Select
Collaborate	Facilitate	Order	Sell
Communicate	Familiarize	Organize	Serve
Compare	Forecast	Originate	Settle
Compile	Formulate	Oversee	Solve
Complete	Generate	Perceive	Speak
Conceive	Govern	Perform	Staff
Conciliate	Guide	Persuade	Standardize
Conduct	Handle	Plan	Stimulate
Consult	Head	Prepare	Summarize
Contract	Hire	Present	Supervise
Control	Identify	Preside	Support
Cooperate	Implement	Process	Survey
Coordinate	Improve	Produce	Synthesize
Correct	Increase	Program	Systematize
Counsel	Index	Promote	Teach
Create	Influence	Propose	Train
Decide	Inform	Provide	

The Clinical Medical Assistant Program

THE INTERVIEW

YOU HAVE 5 MINUTES

That's why first impressions—being on time, being dressed appropriately and being prepared—are critical. If you make a bad first impression, it's going to be a lot harder for you to convince someone to hire you. The interview is the most important aspect of any job hunt. The impression you make on an employer will likely be the reason you get a job offer or not.

As mentioned previously, preparation is the key to any interview. The following guidelines will assist you in presenting a positive first impression:

1. **Look Sharp.**

   Before the interview, select your outfit. Depending on the industry and position, get out your best duds and check them over for spots and wrinkles.

2. **Be on Time.**

   Never arrive late to an interview. Allow extra time to arrive early in the vicinity, allowing for factors like getting lost. Enter the building 10 to 15 minutes before the interview.

3. **Do Your Research.**

   Research the company before the interview. The more you know about the company and what it stands for, the better chance you have of selling yourself.

This "Student Graduate Assistance Packet" and any attachments are the confidential property of Condensed Curriculum International Inc.

D-11

4. **Be Prepared.**

   Bring along a folder containing extra copies of your resume, a copy of your references and paper to take notes. You should also have questions prepared to ask at the end of the interview.

5. **Show Enthusiasm.**

   A firm handshake and plenty of eye contact demonstrate confidence.

6. **Listen.**

   One of the most neglected interviewing skills is *listening*.

7. **Answer the Question Asked.**

   Candidates often don't think about whether or not they actually are answering the questions asked by their interviewers. Make sure you understand what is being asked, and get further clarification if you are unsure.

8. **Give Specific Examples.**

   One specific example of your background is worth 50 vague stories. Prepare your stories before the interview. Give examples that highlight your successes and uniqueness.

9. **Ask Questions.**

   Many interviewees don't ask questions and miss the opportunity to find out valuable information. Your questions indicate your interest in the company or job.

10. **Follow Up.**

    Whether it's through email or regular mail, *the follow-up* is one more chance to remind the interviewer of all the valuable traits you bring to the job and company. You don't want to miss this last chance to market yourself.

INTERVIEWING SKILLS

Sell It to Me, Don't Tell It to Me

Interviews are the time to sell what you have accomplished, not simply to tell what you've done. Be prepared to give examples of your accomplishments to back up you statements. An example of this is: "In my current position I suggested a change in the scheduling which allowed greater utilization of our employees and reduced turn-around-time for our customers by 20%."

This is why it is vital that you practice your responses.

- Think of what questions the interviewer may ask and practice your answers. This will allow you to make sure that your answers are clear and concise and not long-winded.
- Practice will also help to reduce some of your anxiety and increase your confidence level.
- Before the interview, think of your five best strengths. What makes them strengths? Think of examples in your past performance that provides proof of these strengths and what is the best way to convey this information to the person interviewing you.
- Every interview concludes with the interviewer asking if you have any questions. The worst thing to say is that you have no questions. Again be prepared. During your research of the company did any questions arise? Did any of the statements made by the person interviewing you, provide any questions? For example; during your research you learned that the company would be

expanding their outpatient facilities. This would provide an excellent opportunity to show your knowledge and interest in the future growth of the company by inquiring about this expansion.
- Never ask about benefits or salary during the interview process. The time for these questions is when the position has been offered to you.

COMMON INTERVIEW QUESTIONS

1. What are your strengths, assets, and things you do well and like about yourself?

2. What are your shortcomings, weaker points and areas for improvement?

3. Why should I hire you? How can you be an asset to this company?

4. Tell me about yourself.

5. Technical questions related to specific job functions.

6. What is your ideal coworker, supervisor or job environment?

HANDLING ILLEGAL QUESTIONS

Various federal, state, and local laws regulate the questions a prospective employer can ask you, the job candidate. An employer's questions—whether on the job application, in the interview, or during the testing process—must be related to the job you're seeking. For the employer, the focus must be: "What do I need to know to decide whether this person can perform the functions of this job?"

If asked an illegal question, you have three options:

- You can answer the question.
- You can refuse to answer the question, which is well within your rights.
- You can examine the question for its intent and respond with an answer as it might apply to the job. Let's say the interviewer asks, "Who is going to take care of your children when you are at work?" You might answer, "I can meet the work schedule that this job requires."

KEEPING TRACK OF IT ALL!

If you are keeping your promise and meeting the goal you set, you will accumulate quite a bit of data. It is important that all of this information be documented to ensure that you follow up on cold calls, cold visits, interviews etc. in a timely manner. The chart below will assist you in organizing your job search and keeping track of those important contacts.

Job applied for	Company/contact Name	Phone/fax #	Date resume submitted	Follow up dates/comments

The Clinical Medical Assistant Program

INTERVIEW FOLLOW UP

BE PERSISTENT—NOT A PEST

A thank you note or letter is a must when looking for a job. It will set you apart from the crowd as well as provide another opportunity to be front and center in the interviewer's mind.

Your thank you letter should use the same format and presentation as your resume. It should reiterate your skills and your interest in the position being offered.

THE RETURN CALL

If you don't get a return call as promised, call them and leave a message. Be prepared, professional and courteous. Try to reach the person at least once, explaining you want the information before you consider other positions because this company is your first choice. If you don't get an answer, consider it a "No." There is a fine line between being persistent and being a pest.

You may get lucky and actually reach the person when you call. If you do have such luck, use this opportunity to ask for feedback on your interview. Sometimes, not often, a person will take the time to give you advice. If this happens, be grateful and learn from the experience.

This "Student Graduate Assistance Packet" and any attachments are the confidential property of Condensed Curriculum International Inc.

D-15

Name of person
The person's title
Name of company
Address

Date

Dear _____:

It was a pleasure to meet with you to discuss the position of _____.

I am very excited about the chance of becoming a productive member of your team. I am confident that the extensive _____ training I have already received will enable me to represent your company with integrity and skill.

During our discussion, I sensed your strong belief in providing quality service. I want to assure you of my conviction to this important task and I will strive to perform to this standard on a daily basis.

Thank you for this opportunity and I look forward to discussing the next step in the employment process soon.

Respectfully,

The Clinical Medical Assistant Program

THE JOB SEARCH

WHERE DO I START?

Looking for employment is a full time job! Tough times call for tough strategies. Take the time to sit down and create a strategy including a commitment to call, mail a resume, or visit two places of employment a minimum of three days each week. Searching for a job can be discouraging and it's important that you set goals and stick with them!

- Go through the telephone book and make a list of every facility in your area that employs your qualifications
- Network with your family and friends and let everyone know you are looking for a job
- Call your references and let them know that you will be giving out their name again. No references lined up? Get some!
- Create or update your resume

COLD CALLS

If you find that your networking prospects are drying up, it may be time to think of new ways to penetrate the job market. The cold call is a basic technique used in selling, and when done properly, it

This "Student Graduate Assistance Packet" and any attachments are the confidential property of Condensed Curriculum International Inc.

D-17

can provide new opportunities for you. If the very thought of calling a stranger and selling yourself makes you cringe, you are not alone.

- Preparing a script to read from before making the call.
- Begin with a greeting—sounding enthusiastic (but not phony) will be a plus. Introduce yourself and say what your specialty is and how many years of experience you have in your field or any training you have received.
- Ask the magic question, 'When can I come in for an interview?"

Not everyone you call will be interested in what you're selling. Expect rejection; two out of every three calls will not lead to new prospects. But success is the result of trying. Your career will benefit from determination and consistent effort.

When looking for employment, persistence is the key. It is hard work but once you find that dream job it will be all worth the blood, sweat and yes those tears!

HOW FLEXIBLE ARE YOU?

Today's companies are seeking employees that possess not only the knowledge to perform multiple duties but also the willingness to multitask. The rising cost of healthcare requires that job functions be diverse and multifunctional. Candidates that show an interest in learning a new skill, performing several job functions, or working various shifts are much more attractive to the potential employer than someone not willing to bend in difficult times. Often positions are offered internally to current employees. Today's candidates need to be flexible. This may require a person to take a position that is less desirable in order to be eligible to apply for the preferred position once they are an employee.

According to the Bureau of Labor Statistics . . .

"Health care will generate 3 million new wage and salary jobs between 2008 and 2016, more than any other industry."

As the largest industry in 2006, health care provided 14 million jobs—13.6 million jobs for wage and salary workers and about 438,000 jobs for the self-employed. Also, 7 of the 20 fastest growing occupations are health care related. Most workers have jobs that require less than 4 years of college education, but health diagnosing and treating practitioners are among the most educated workers.

"ONCE I HAVE THE SKILLS, WHERE CAN I USE THEM?"

Public Hospitals	Primary Care Office
Medical Clinic	Private Hospitals
Rehab Hospital	Clinical laboratory
Independent Laboratory	Cardiology Practice
Hospital Pharmacy	Out Patient Rehab
Urgent Care Clinic	Multi-physician's Office
Home Health Care	Out Patient Laboratory
Hospice	Insurance Companies
Independent Pharmacy	Research Facility
Long-term-care Facilities	HMOs
Pharmaceutical Supply Company	Ambulatory Care Centers
Out Patient Surgery Center	Billing Company
Occupational Health	Radiology Facilities

Specialist's Office
Psychiatric Facility
VA Hospital
Pediatric Centers
Public Health Department
Chronic Care Facility
Physical Therapy Clinic
Medical Record Department

Ophthalmologist's Office
Acute Care Hospital
Cancer Centers
Birthing Center
Red Cross
Blood Banks
Sports Medicine Facility
Skilled Nursing Facility